SUPERNOURISHMENT

for Children with Autism Spectrum Disorder

SUPERNOURISHMENT

for Children with Autism Spectrum Disorder

A Practical Nutritional Approach to Optimizing
Diet for Whole Brain and Body Health

ANGELETTE MÜLLER

Jessica Kingsley *Publishers*
London and Philadelphia

First published in 2016
by Jessica Kingsley Publishers
73 Collier Street
London N1 9BE, UK
and
400 Market Street, Suite 400
Philadelphia, PA 19106, USA

www.jkp.com

Library of Congress Cataloging in Publication Data
Müller, Angelette.
  Supernourishment for children with autism spectrum
disorder : a practical nutritional approach to
optimizing diet for whole brain and body health / Angelette Müller.
     pages cm
  Includes bibliographical references and index.
  ISBN 978-1-84905-383-9 (alk. paper)
 1. Autism spectrum disorders in children--Alternative treatment. I. Title.
  RJ506.A9M86 2016
  618.92'85882--dc23
                          2015010025

British Library Cataloguing in Publication Data
A CIP catalogue record for this book is available from the British Library

ISBN 978 1 84905 383 9
eISBN 978 0 85700 746 9

Printed and bound in China

To Creator God
Thank you for making us so wonderfully,
and packing us and food with so much potential.

To the health professionals
Who have influenced my knowledge journey.

To my family
To my family and Mother Georgina and daughter Zayne
for prayers, support and inspiration.

To the families
To all the families that I have worked with who work tirelessly to help their
children. Thank you for giving me the opportunity to learn alongside you.

To the little heroes
The children with autism
who amazingly navigate life from such a young age
with all its unique challenges in such a brave and courageous way.

Thank you.

DISCLAIMERS

This book is intended as a guide with the main aim of promoting the nutritional density of the diet. Each child is unique. If you suspect allergies or sensitivities to foods, seek guidance from physicians or licensed health professionals.

The nutritional adequacy of a diet is important, especially for growing children. Any dietary manipulation that would require complete exclusion of a food group requires support from licensed health professionals, as children are particularly vulnerable to nutrient deficiencies as they are still growing.

None of this advice replaces medical recommendations.

Note that all names used within the text have been changed to protect the privacy of the individuals.

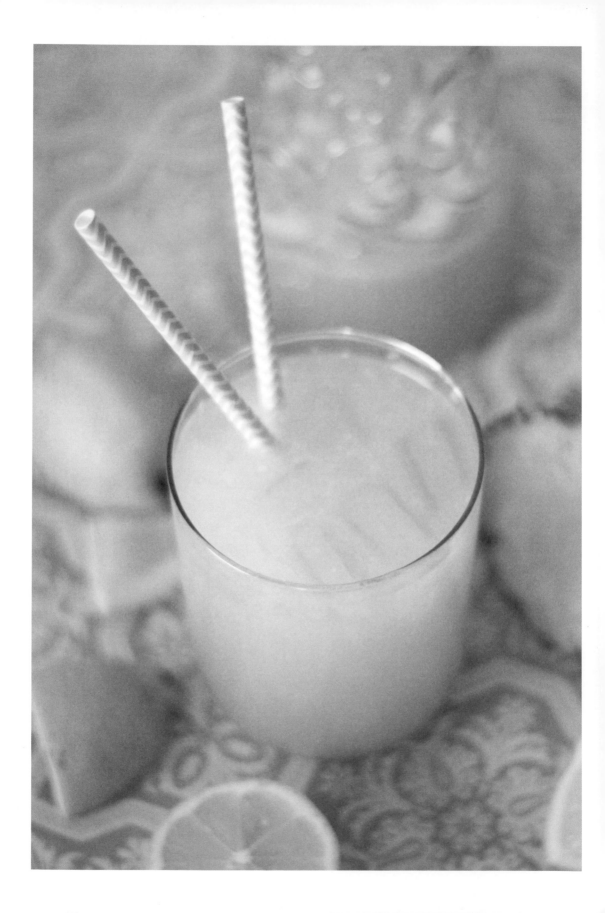

CONTENTS

ABBREVIATIONS

CF   Casein free

FODMAP   Fermentable, oligo-, di-, monosaccharides and polyol

GAPS   Gut and Psychology Syndrome

GF   Gluten free

GI   Glycaemic index

GL   Glycaemic load

RDA   Recommended daily allowance

SCD   Specific carbohydrate diet

Introduction

The Whole Child Health Approach

We know the answers to many questions about the mind and body, but there arc some questions that we are struggling to answer. Why does a six-year-old boy entering the clinic room cower in the corner, away from the adults, only to return to the clinic after six weeks on a modified diet to interact playfully with the people in the room, 'as though a light bulb has been turned on' (parent's comment on the change in the child)? Why does a toddler who is having big challenges with speech start to talk after one week of dietary modification? Or why does a five-year-old boy who displays consistent aggressive behaviour calm down after his diet is changed? I know we have ideas and explanations for some of these changes, but we know many answers are right at the cusp of the newest research. We know a lot about how the body and mind works, but we are still learning how to integrate the complicated web of interactions that allow the human mind and body to function, just like the complex coordination of the brain and the body that allows for understanding what someone is saying. In order to understand a spoken instruction we need to have enough energy for both the processing speed required and for the co-ordination of brain rhythms.

This books attempts to look a little more closely at diet. It emphasizes the importance of a wholefood diet with the spectrum of all its natural nutrients to help to protect and provide the functions needed for the mind and body of a child. We look at the ideas behind why diet may not work, and why it can work. This is followed by practical recipes, which are simple to make, to increase the nutritional density of the diet. In this way we hope the recipes will provide supernourishment for the whole child.

HOW TO USE
THE BOOK

Part I provides the background, looking at the possible links between diet, brain, symptoms and behaviour in children with autism. It begins by looking at some of the reasons why children respond differently to their diet being modified. Understanding how an overly processed diet can lead to a depletion of nutrients sets the stage to understand why we need to supernourish the diet with natural, minimally processed foods. Many children with autism also have sensitivities or allergies that are often driven by poor digestion, imbalances in gut flora and problems breaking down and eliminating certain substances. We look at each food group, highlighting some of these issues to raise awareness of how ingredients in foods can be an issue for people with certain types of food sensitivities.

Part II looks at the practical side. There are simple, supernourishing recipes for breakfasts, lunches, evening meals, snacks and drinks. We know that many children with autism follow a specific dietary modification, and each recipe has a grid to show which diets the recipe complies with.

This is then followed by Part III, which contains advice about meal and menu planning. The final chapter is aimed at helping parents/clinicians to be aware of some of the challenges that children may face that could contribute to problem eating.

PART I
NUTRITION, NOURISHMENT AND AUTISM

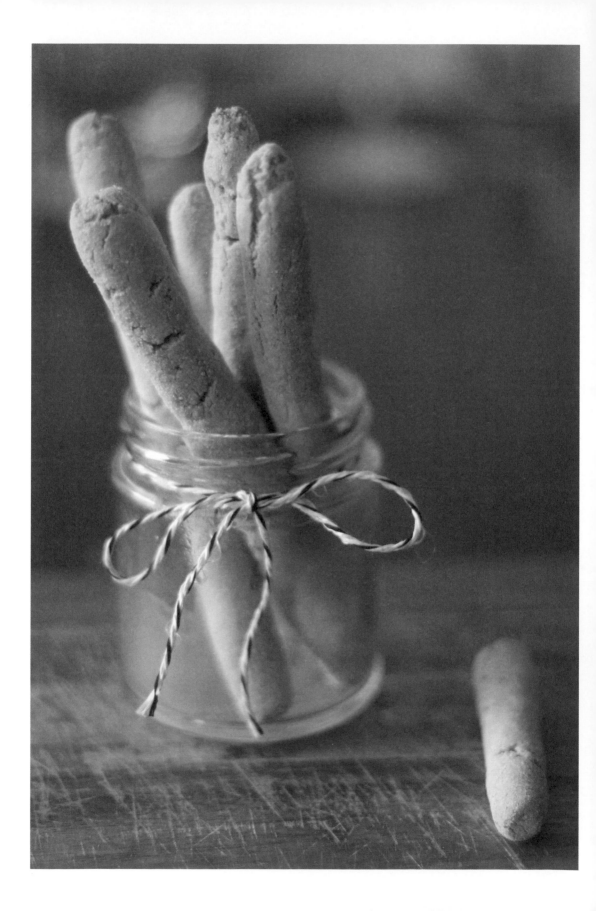

1 Brain, Behaviour, Bugs and Diet

I have worked with hundreds of families to help them modify the diet of their child with autism. At the beginning of my journey I knew diet could make an impact on health. After all, the food we eat makes up the literal building blocks of our body. But I had no idea about the potential effect diet could have on behaviour.

At the clinic we would always assess how children were responding to the diet. Sometimes we would ask the parents to report any changes they saw. Or we would use questionnaires, such as the Childhood Autism Rating Scale (CARS), a questionnaire that uses a scale to rate a child's behaviour by observing how they relate to different things such as interaction with people, responses to what they see, hear, taste or touch, and how they adapt to change or communicate. Other times we would use video recording with permission from the parents, and observe the differences in behaviour and communication before and after the diet. We also used a variety of tests. Most parents reported improvements after trying the dietary changes, and we saw differences when looking back at the videos, and positive improvements when reviewing the testing.

It was exciting to see these positive changes and reports. But it was not until I met Raymond that I was fully convinced of the power of diet to impact behaviour. We had been working with Raymond for about three months. He was following a gluten- and casein-free diet. His parents had noted improvements in his eye contact, concentration and language, but there were still many challenges.

Raymond had come into the clinic for a clinical review. Our clinic room was lit up with little mushroom lights that gave the room a subtle glow. When

Raymond arrived, he was watching YouTube videos on his iPad. We asked his dad to take away the iPad so we could see how he would respond. Raymond was not happy. He gave us a full display of his displeasure. Mushroom lights flew through the air and toy lorries skidded across the polished floor. His little fists began to fly in every direction.[1]

Raymond was already on a gluten- and casein-free diet. He was also taking supplements. We scratched our heads a little. Gluten and dairy exclusion had already been a big change for the family. Since beginning the diet they had reported improvements in language, eye contact and understanding, but he was still experiencing regular outbursts as well as other behaviour challenges. We managed to complete the consultation, and recommend a natural diet where most of the food is homemade, and processed carbohydrates and specific starchy foods are replaced with lower carbohydrate vegetables.[2]

Four weeks later Raymond was back. To our surprise, he was sitting quietly at the table with his dad, communicating in words mixed with soft tones. He was interacting calmly. We challenged Raymond by taking his iPad away. There was not even a tiny protest. His parents reported positive changes at home as well. They had followed the diet strictly for four weeks. They attributed the positive changes in Raymond to the diet.

How could diet have made such a difference? We came to realize that the answers to this simple question were quite complex.

The Brain, Gut and Behaviour Connections

How can food, the gut and the brain affect behaviour? We know that one of the main ways that the gut talks to the brain is via a special nerve known as the vagus nerve. This nerve wanders around the body and is dedicated to sending information back to the brain. It dedicates a surprising percentage of its hotline space for messages to be sent from the gut to the brain. It also sends brain messages back down to the gut. These messages can affect the movement of the gut, speeding up transit (diarrhoea) or slowing it down (constipation). Its rhythms of information can also affect digestion, increasing or decreasing enzyme release. Its gentle pulses even affect overall gut health through helping the gut lining stay healthy or breaking it down.[3]

The vagus nerve's sensing activities allow it to detect every aspect of the food we eat, sensing both nutrient and non-nutrient intake. It can assess the size and shape of the food, the chemicals in the food, and anything else that comes in with food. It then has a conversation with the brain to decide how to respond. The response may include activation of the immune system or pain receptors or any other response deemed appropriate.[4]

Vagus Nerve and Autism

Interestingly, most of the research about the vagus nerve relates to its effect on social behaviour. Stimulation of the vagus nerve releases oxytocin, a brain protein associated with bonding and social behaviour. Oxytocin has been looked at in a lot of detail in relation to autism.

But how could the complex brain–gut conversations affect behaviour? We really are just beginning to find out. In the area of behaviour and the gut, little mice offer us some clues. I know it might be hard to imagine that a mouse can display anxiety-like behaviour, but researchers believe they do. And one of the things that promotes anxiety-like behaviour is poorly digested carbohydrates.[5] We also see similar patterns of sugar affecting mental well-being in humans, where they might be more prone to depression if they have problems breaking down the fruit sugar fructose. Yes, it is a bit of a leap, but a leap that is generating intense interest from scientists. It is much more than just the gut and brain that researchers are looking at. It is a huge community with trillions of cells. These tiny bugs are known as the gut microbiome, 'micro' meaning 'small' and 'biome' meaning 'a naturally occurring place where either plants or animals live'. In this case, the 'biome' is made up of trillions of bugs like bacteria, yeasts, fungi, viruses and bacterial-like mini-bugs known as archaea.

What Are Gut Flora?

Gut flora are the population of bacteria, viruses, yeasts and archaea (very similar to bacteria) that normally live in the gut. There are trillions of these micro-organisms, and changes to diet and other factors such as stress, antibiotics or infections, can create an imbalance in the flora community. Gut flora are sometimes called microbiota in the research.

And it's the way these bugs behave in response to our diet and other environmental factors that may hold a clue to explain why the gut and brain may be able to impact behaviour.

Much has been said on major gut issues in the area of autism. Different research papers say different things, some suggesting that there is no relationship between increased gut problems and autism, and others saying that there is up to a 90 per cent increase in gut issues with autism. In clinic we could not help noticing that many children who attend the clinic experience gut-related issues, such as constipation, diarrhoea, bloating, flatulence, undigested foods in their stools, abdominal discomfort or pain or reflux. I also found it difficult to ignore the observation that with a change of diet, some of these symptoms are alleviated, with improvements in behaviours, such as sleep, concentration and communication.

Again, it begs the question: Why would dietary changes help to improve behaviours? I wonder if we can say that at least a sub-group of children with autism have an increased risk of gut-related issues, one of which is related to poor carbohydrate digestion. We know from research that digestive ability is compromised in some children with autism. One of the reasons for this is that their body is not producing enough digestive enzymes to break down foods in the gut. Williams and colleagues from the Center for Infection and Immunity, Columbia University, New York,[6] reported that some children with autism have lower levels of enzymes to break down carbohydrates. They also seemed to lack transporters, protein-like tubes that usher the carbohydrates from the gut into the body. Poor digestion means more 'food' is sitting around in the gut, resulting in gut bugs feasting on these bits of undigested food, which leads to an overgrowth of bugs in the small intestine. This overgrowth of bugs and the resulting fermenting foods leads to water being drawn into the gut (osmosis), with possible symptoms of diarrhoea. Excess production of gases is another symptom, which leads to bloating, flatulence and abdominal discomfort.

What Is a Digestive Enzyme?

Digestive enzymes are active proteins that speed up the breakdown of food in the process of digestion. For example, potato crisps are rich in carbohydrates. Digesting potato crisps requires enzymes to break up the long chains of sugars into single sugars like glucose for absorption.

The bugs themselves also have an influence on the brain. They can send substances into the brain, influencing the physiological 'decisions' made. They can also send lots of 'chatter', sending messages via the vagus nerve and brainstem to the brain. You could compare it to ten people trying to talk to you all at once – it can get quite frustrating. As you can imagine, it might not just be your brainstem that gets irritable. You might get irritated yourself, affecting your behaviour.

This may sound far-fetched, but I imagine that the more we learn about gut bugs, the more we will learn about behaviour. And maybe we will have a least a little more insight as to how Raymond became so much calmer after changing the types of carbohydrates he ate.

Of course it would be wonderful if there was one explanation for why children with autism behave the way they do, but we know that it's really not that simple. There seems to be no end to the possible reasons that play a role in increasing risk or severity of autism.

In this chapter we look at a bit of the history of how we came to know about autism. And we touch briefly on the challenge we face in understanding autism within the medical model. We then take a closer look at the many ways that diet can impact the way the body functions, and how this can then affect the brain and maybe even behaviours.

Emerging Mind/Body Understanding

It's no surprise that we find it difficult to see relationships between mind and body health. After all, René Descartes, philosopher and mathematician, was quite convincing when he presented the idea that the mind and body were two different 'substances'. We can even guess from the word 'substances' that at that stage in history (the 16th century) we really didn't get it. We just did not know enough about the body and mind to draw conclusions about the relationships between them.

Fast forward to the 20th century. It's the early 1940s, and Leo Kanner, psychiatrist, is working at Johns Hopkins University (Kanner was known as the 'father of child psychiatry' in the US). He carefully describes the behaviour of 11 children and uses the word 'autistic'.[7] Autism, taken from the Latin word *autos* (meaning self), was borrowed from Eugene Bleuer, Swiss psychiatrist. In order to understand the time context, Bleuer was the first person to define schizophrenia, and he used the word 'autism' to describe the withdrawal from relationships he observed in schizophrenics.[8] At this time there was no diagnostic criteria for autism. It was not until 1952, when the first edition of the *Diagnostic and Statistical Manual of Mental Disorders* (DSM) was published,[9] that autism was classified within childhood schizophrenia. Later, in 1980, following the seminal work of the first British child psychiatrist Sir Michael Rutter, autism was distinguished from childhood schizophrenia and given its own distinct category.[10]

So psychiatry was in its infancy, and it was not alone. Knowledge of physiology was on a parallel journey. We were just learning more about the brain and physiology. Understandably we would not have made the links between a neurodevelopmental condition such as autism with something physiological such as serotonin and autism. Would we have been able to make links between genetics and autism when we were still working out the basic structure of genetic material (DNA, deoxyribonucleic acid)?[11]

Almost 50 years after the first DSM was produced, an admission was made. We had found out more about the brain and the body, and were struggling to maintain the dividing line between mind and body, mental disorders and physical imbalances. In 1994, in the fourth edition of the DSM (DSM-IV),[12] we outlined the struggle: 'The term mental disorder unfortunately implies a distinction between "mental" disorders and "physical" disorders… there is much "physical" in "mental" disorders and much "mental" in "physical" disorders.'[13]

The research had begun to catch up. We knew that the artificial dividing line between brain and body was fading away.

Disease and the Mind

This dividing line between mind and body had influenced the way we defined disease in a big way. This then impacted the way we treated disease. In his book, *How Scientists Explain Disease*, Paul Thagard[14] explains that when we think about physical disorders or disease, we label the disease according to system location (e.g. cardiovascular disease), nutritional deficiencies (e.g. scurvy and vitamin C) or infectious agents (e.g. Helicobacter pylori).

But was such a division reflecting what the research was showing us about mental/developmental and physical disorders? Links between system disorders like heart disease, infections or even nutritional imbalances were becoming more associated with mental health issues. People with schizophrenia were twice as likely to experience heart disease.[15] Infections with viruses or bacteria like cytomegalovirus (a virus from the herpes group) and chlamydia trachomatis (bacteria) were associated with increased risk of schizophrenia.[16] Symptoms such as hallucinations and delusions were reported as improving in some patients after introducing a gluten-free diet.[17]

Autism showed similar patterns. People with autism have a higher risk of developing coronary heart disease. Infections, both prenatally and during early infancy, were linked with autism. Strangely there are also reports of viral infections being associated with autistic-like behaviours in both older children and in adults. One case study describes a 14-year-old girl who developed the classical symptoms of autism over a 70-day period following an infection.[18] Another describes a man who developed autistic-like symptoms following the development of herpes encephalitis (a condition where the brain becomes inflamed secondary to herpes infection).[19] Different studies also point to the beneficial effect of diet and specific nutrients in some children with autism.[20]

Can Diet Help?

This leads us to ask: If infections increase the risk of 'system' diseases and nutritional issues, could they also play a role in mental or neurodevelopmental conditions? Is there a chance that changing the diet, for example, can have a positive impact on the health outcome? For example, a reduction in some symptoms or behaviours? Could diet positively impact autism?

There is plenty of debate and controversy surrounding this question of diet. To gain a better understanding I thought we could look at one specific diet in relation to autism. We will use the gluten- and casein-free diet, mainly because it is the most well-researched diet for autism and possibly the most popular.

The gluten- and casein-free diet is a diet that excludes gluten and casein. Gluten is a stringy set of proteins that helps give wheat-based bread its stretchy characteristics, and is present in barley, rye and some oats. Casein is a complex protein found in milk of dairy origin and all of its products (e.g. cheese, cream and yoghurt).

Cochrane reviews are well-respected and are 'internationally recognized as the highest standard of evidence-based health care'. In 2008 they produced a paper entitled 'Gluten- and casein-free diets for autistic spectrum disorder'.[21] In this they reviewed various studies looking at the effects of either the gluten- or casein-free diet, or a combination of a gluten- and casein-free diet. Improvements in some of the following symptoms were noted:

- communication and use of language

- attention and concentration

- social integration and interaction

- self-injurious behaviour/altered pain perception

- repetitive or stereotyped patterns of behaviour

- motor coordination

- hyperactivity

- functional bowel disorders (e.g. diarrhoea, constipation)

- epilepsy and seizure-type disorders.

Nor all the papers reported positive changes. And the Cochrane paper concluded that there was 'lack of evidence to support the use of the gluten and casein free diet', and more research was needed.[22]

Why are there so many differences of opinion about whether the GF/CF diet works? And can dietary changes help children with autism? I wonder if some of the confusion about whether or not dietary change is beneficial may stem from the large degree of variation in why a child may or may not respond to the dietary change. Different approaches may be needed depending on each child's unique needs.

Table 1.1 shows some explanations for why a gluten- or dairy-free diet might be beneficial for a subgroup of patients, and the background for these explanations. There are also example of symptoms that are sometimes attributed to these explanations or conditions. The table illustrates that there are numerous causes that can contribute to the potential range of symptoms observed in children with autism.

The speed of response to dietary exclusion of a specific food may vary between children; and there may be no response at all if eating a specific food does not pose a problem for the child. For example, constipation is a classic symptom of cow's milk allergy but there are other explanations for constipation as a response to cow's milk ingestion, 'opioid excess' being one of them. The opioid excess theory was first suggested by Jaak Panksepp, professor of psychology and a neuroscientist. He first noticed similarities between the effects of low doses of narcotic drugs (that contained opioids) and autistic-like behaviours.[23] Opioids are protein shapes that are present in plants and foods (e.g. poppies, wheat and dairy). Medication such as morphine also contains opioids. The opioid excess theory suggests that children with increased gut permeability (where bigger proteins pass from the gut to the system) may be more sensitive to the presence of opioids. Some people believe that constipation can be relieved in children with autism by removing foods that certain opoid-like substances. If we remove dairy from the diet and some children become constipated while others do not, a reasonable conclusion would be that the dairy-free diet is not always effective.

As dietary requirements begin to emerge, it's important to consider whether other foods may needs to be removed from the diet. In 'opioid excess theory', for example, high-opioid-like protein foods such as wheat, bread, crackers and wheat pasta also need to be removed to see an obvious response. Or imagine if we remove dairy, such as cow's milk and yoghurt, only to replace it with the dairy-free alternative soya milk. If the child is sensitive both to cow's milk and soy milk, would we notice a positive response? Maybe not. What if the child has no sensitivities or allergies to cow's milk or its products – would we see any positive changes when removing dairy from the diet? Probably not.

These many reasons illustrate how difficult it can be to interpret a child's response to dietary change. We also have to acknowledge that not all dietary alternatives are equally nutritious. If we use the gluten-free diet as an example, gluten-free products are often highly refined. This might mean a greater level of overall carbohydrate intake. Gluten-free toast, for example, has 25 per cent more carbohydrate content than toast made from wholemeal bread. If a highly processed carbohydrate-rich gluten-free diet was given to a child with poor carbohydrate digestion or small intestine bacterial overgrowth, what sort of response might we expect to see? Possibly no difference at all, or even a worsening of symptoms.[24] Or if a child has a greater severity of health issues, for example, chronic infection, poor energy production or inflammation, could this affect responses to dietary changes? Possibly.

Small Intestine Bacterial Overgrowth

This is where bacteria grow to abnormally large numbers – more than should be present in the small intestine – leading to bloating and flatulence.

Children with autism are often more sensitive to environmental factors too. I have seen children's behaviour deteriorate with a change in the seasons, such as when there is an increase in pollen during springtime, if a child has pollen sensitivity, or a worsening of symptoms or behaviour after a viral infection such as the flu, or when staying in a damp/mouldy house.

These examples show us the complexity we face when looking at how dietary changes affect children with autism. This highlights the need to look at the many factors coming together to influence the effects of dietary change or behavioural/symptomatic changes, such as quality of food choices within a diet, underlying issues such as lactose intolerance or allergies, the health of the child, and the child's environment that may overlap to present a more complex picture.

We also need to consider the effects of excluding specific foods from the diet and how this will affect the overall nutritional adequacy of the diet, and recognize that different children may have different levels of nutritional needs depending on their health or genetic predisposition.

In light of this, it may be easier to suggest principles for modifying the diet, rather than rules. This should help to ensure that any changes promote the supernourishment of the child.

Table 1.1: Factors that may explain why a gluten- and casein-free diet can work

Condition	How does it work?	Symptoms
Gluten sensitivity	Gluten sensitivity (GS) may occur six times more frequently than coeliac disease. Antibodies (immune proteins that alert the body to foreign substances) are made into gliadin, which is a component of gluten. Symptoms associated with GS are listed in the next column.[25]	Abdominal pain Constipation Chronic diarrhoea Bloating Vomiting Headache Tiredness Limb pain Failure to thrive
Food allergy	Eating casein/dairy products can result in non-immunoglobulin E (IgE) mediated cow's milk protein allergy. A history of colic and vomiting is seen in early infancy, and diarrhoea and loose stools in older children.[26]	Diarrhoea Bloating Abdominal cramp Constipation
Food intolerance	Lactose intolerance occurs when there is not enough of the milk-digesting enzyme lactase. The severity of the symptoms depends on the level of lactase deficiency and amount of milk sugars eaten. A fructan is a short chain of fructose (fruit sugar) present in larger amounts in various foods including products containing gluten. People with fructan intolerance may have small intestine bacterial overgrowth, inflammation of the gut, lower levels of enzymes and transporters as well as habits such as gulping down food.[27]	Diarrhoea Stomach cramps Stomach rumbling Nausea Bloating Flatulence Indigestion

Intestinal barrier integrity	There is a significant association between compromised gut permeability and children with autism.[28]	Various gut-related symptoms
Antibodies to Purkinje cells in cerebellum	Immune proteins called antibodies can fight against gluten and casein. Some children with autism have greater level of these antibodies. These antibodies appear to promote inflammation and damage special cells called Purkinje cells involved in movement and coordination.[29]	Motor coordination
Opioid excess	During digestion, gluten and casein are broken down into smaller protein units called peptides. These little proteins have opioid activity. Casein in cow's milk opioid is bovine beta-casein yielding beta-casomorphin-7; and in gluten, alpha-gliadin, giving rise to gliadinomorphin-7. These little proteins can act on the opioid receptors. Opioids are involved in brain development, pain management, gut motility and constipation. The opioid excess theory suggests that children with autism have a greater degree of gut permeability. This means that partially undigested proteins can pass from the gut into body, from the body to the brain.[30]	Self-injurious behaviour Pain perception Eye contact Constipation
Bacterial lipopoly-saccharides	Increased gut permeability means proteins in the gut can be transported between the cells into the system. This would include 'coats' (outer cell wall) shed from gut bacteria known as lipopolysaccharides (LPS). This allows LPS to enter the body's circulation and to promote brain and body inflammation.[31]	Any symptom associated with potential effects of inflammation (systemic and brain)
Impact on nutrient absorption	This can be made worse because both gluten and casein lower cysteine uptake, cysteine being one of the building blocks of glutathione. Lower levels of glutathione possibly contribute to inflammation.[32]	Any effect of poor nutrient including antioxidant absorption

2 Why Wholefoods Are So Important

I remember looking at the food diary. Three foods – cornflakes, yoghurt and rice cakes. It amazed me to see that a five-year-old boy could survive on only three foods. Another child, two foods – eggs and rice. How did his body manage? In both cases, each child's diet was severely restricted, but the children seemed to be surviving, growing and looking well. The ability of our bodies to function on limited dietary resources shows the amazing resilience of the human body.

But the body is not always this successful. We read about stories such as a five-year-old boy who developed an open sore on his eye due to vitamin A deficiency after living off two foods – bacon and muffins – and drinking only Kool-Aid®, although I am sure that he was nutritionally deficient for quite some time before he developed such a glaring symptom. And of course the two boys I saw in clinic on the limited diet also showed nutritional deficiencies on testing.

Nutritional deficiency is a main concern, and we observe it frequently in the children who attend clinic. Various deficiencies include vitamin D, magnesium, B vitamins (especially vitamin B2), omega-3 fatty acids and various mineral deficiencies. Often many of the children with these deficiencies appear healthy, but it is not until they start following a healthier diet and sometimes with supplementation that their nutrient levels improve, and parents have reported positive outcomes, such as improved immune function, more energy, less hyperactivity, better concentration and better eye contact in their children.

Although our body will make a brave attempt to compensate for a given nutrient deficiency, our main dietary goals are to improve the diet so that the body does not have to compensate in this way. Instead, we want to provide nutrient-packed food so that the body can function at its full potential.

Looking More Closely at Dietary Patterns

When parents attend the clinic, they complete a food diary listing typical foods eaten at breakfast, lunch, evening meal, snacks, as well as drinks. They also complete a list of all foods eaten including every type of fruit, vegetable, grain, nut, protein source, sugary food and oil. From this information we look at the general pattern of food intake. Children arriving at clinic for the first time are frequently following a restricted and/or overly processed diet.

In this section we review the patterns in food intake for starchy carbohydrates, fruits and vegetables, proteins, fats, dairy, drinks and snacks, and consider the nutrients likely to be lacking when foods from the food group are processed, or when low levels of the food are eaten. We also think about the impact this could have on the diet, if the intake of nutrients is lower.

At the end of this chapter we look at energy production as an example of how nutrients work together in synergy. By showing this example we hope to illustrate the importance of eating a variety of natural wholefoods, rich in a whole spectrum of nutrients, instead of highly processed food choices.

Starchy Carbohydrates

Starchy carbohydrates include cereals, pastas, potatoes, breads, crackers, grains or pseudo-grains (grains that are similar to grains, but that are not classified as a grain, such as quinoa). This group of foods tends to contain high levels of carbohydrates compared to other food groups, with up to 70–90 per cent of carbohydrates (these starchy carbohydrates are simply long chains of sugars).

Breakfast

At breakfast the pattern for a typical dietary intake includes starchy carbohydrates such as Weetabix®, Rice Krispies® or cornflakes, toast or bread, with both wheat-based and gluten-free breads used, usually white gluten-free or wheat-based, or very sweet choices, such as cookies or biscuits.

Lunch/Evening Meal

Typical lunchtime and evening meals follow a similar pattern of highly processed carbohydrates. This includes white rice, pasta dishes such as spaghetti Bolognese, lasagne, pasta shapes and tomato sauce, white flour products such as pizzas or pies, and white bread sandwiches or chips (fries).

Table 2.1: Nutritional values of a range of starchy carbohydrate-containing foods

Food name	Quantity (g)	Energy (Kcal)	Carb.	Starch	Fibre	Sugars
Crispy rice cereal	100	378	84	75	1.5	9.7
Oats, rolled	100	401	73	73	10.5	0
Quinoa flakes	100	379	75	73	7	2.4
Wheat-based cereal biscuits (e.g. Weetabix®)	100	352	76	71	10.9	4.9
Brown rice, boiled	100	141	32	32	1.5	0.5
Pasta twists, white, dried, cooked	100	145	33	32	2.6	0.6
White rice, easy cook, boiled	100	138	31	31	0.8	0
Potato wedges, cooked (oven-baked)	100	209	31	30	4.3	0.9
Spaghetti, wholewheat, dried, cooked	100	132	28	28	4.2	0.1
Potatoes mashed with butter	100	102	15.5	14.6	1.2	0.9
New potatoes in skins, boiled in salted water	100	66	15.4	14.4	1.6	1

Source: Nutritics Professional Dietary Analysis Software (2014).

From the pattern of highly processed carbohydrates that are typically eaten, we can see that the carbohydrate loading can be quite high. Table 2.1 shows that with increased processing, carbohydrate concentration increases. Processing also reduces fibre levels. If we compare two types of rice, a sugary rice cereal with minimally processed brown rice, we would find that 100g of brown rice contains 32g of carbohydrate compared with 84g in the rice cereal. That is more than twice the amount of carbohydrate. A child with compromised carbohydrate digestion should theoretically be able to tolerate the lower carbohydrate option, brown rice, better. However, if the child does not chew their food well, making the brown rice into a porridge for breakfast could be an option, or into pancakes. Either way, by choosing the lower processed form of carbohydrate, we are helping to retain most of the nutrition without having unnecessarily concentrated forms of carbohydrate.

Another example is given for a lunchtime option in Table 2.2 below. Simply replacing a processed carbohydrate-rich choice such as bread and rice cakes with a wholegrain like basmati rice resulted in a 50 per cent reduction in total carbohydrate content. Reducing carbohydrate content in a meal is associated with total calorie reduction. This energy loss can be replaced by adding in a nutrient-dense food such as avocado. Additional options could be replacing bread with a brown rice pancake that could be used as a wrap for the chicken and avocado (see the Egg-Free Fermented Rice Pancakes recipe in Chapter 4).

These examples show us that highly processed carbohydrates tend to have a higher level of total carbohydrates and lower levels of fibre. Higher concentrations of carbohydrate could overload the carbohydrate-digesting capacity of a child. Over time, with poor digestion, this pattern of eating highly processed carbohydrates could lead to increased imbalances of gut flora and symptoms of bloating and flatulence.

Lower fibre levels due to processing food is a concern for a number of reasons. First, fibre helps to regulate blood sugar. Low-fibre cereals with high sugar content can promote blood sugar rises, followed by dips. Low blood sugar levels are often accompanied by symptoms of fatigue, low mood, problems concentrating, and even difficulties in speech. Tantrums can result from the body's attempt to raise blood sugar levels through producing the stress hormone cortisol. High blood sugar can, in turn, lead to hyperactive behaviour. Children with autism can be particularly vulnerable to these types of symptoms. Changing breakfast to a higher fibre, wholefood-based meal with protein results in improvements in many children.

Table 2.2: Nutritional value of certain meals

Food name	Qty (g)	Energy (Kcal)	Carb.	Protein	Fat	Fibre	Sugars
Meal 1	**Ham sandwich, apple, rice cakes**						
Apple, eating (raw)	67	31	7.9	0.3	0.1	1.4	7.9
Rice cakes	18	60	13	1.3	0.6	0.9	0.2
Sandwich, ham, salad, white bread	180	301	45	14.8	8.1	2.3	4.5
Meal total		392	65.9	16.4	8.8	4.6	12.6
Meal 2	**Chicken and rice salad**						
Brown rice, basmati (boiled)	100	114	28	2.3	0.2	0.6	5.5
Carrots, raw	120	42	9.5	0.7	0.4	3.1	8.9
Chicken fillet breast, grilled (small breast)	90	133	0	29	2	0	0
Avocado (¼)	55	104	1	1.2	10.6	2.6	0.3
Meal total		393	39.5	33.2	13.2	6.3	14.7

Source: Nutritics Professional Dietary Analysis Software (2014).

Nutrients

Starchy carbohydrates such as grains in their natural form can be a rich source of nutrients. But when they are processed, there is a major loss of these nutrients. Vitamins B and E are lost, together with plant nutrients and fibre.

Table 2.3 shows selected examples of nutrients lost in the refining process of highly processed carbohydrates like breads and white potatoes. It also lists the possible impact of these lost nutrients on the way the body functions, and potential symptoms that could arise due to deficiencies in these specific nutrients.

We can see from Table 2.3 that refining flour removes most of the B vitamins including B1, B2, B3, B5 and folate. All these B vitamins are involved in different stages of energy production. Low B vitamins can result in lower energy production, affecting the function of both the body and the brain.

Vitamin E is also reduced in refined carbohydrates. This vitamin likes to sit in the cell membrane, the fatty fluid boundary that protects every cell. It normally protects the membrane by stopping tiny high energy 'fires' from changing the shapes of fats and proteins in the membrane, keeping it fluid and flexible. This fluidity helps nutrients to pass into the cell and water to pass out. In this way vitamin E acts as an antioxidant. An antioxidant is a nutrient that is produced inside the body or comes in through the diet to help quench 'oxidative stress', a process that causes damage to the cells and compromises their function. Oxidative stress is also associated with many disease processes and ageing.

Table 2.3: Highly processed carbohydrates and potential loss of nutrients

Typical food choices	Nutrients lost via refining	Functional impact	Symptoms/outcomes
Breakfast Highly processed cereals Gluten-free cereals Gluten-free toast **Lunch/ evening meal** Pasta White rice White potatoes	Refining flour reduces vitamins: B1 (77%), B2 (80%), B3 (81%), B5 (50%) B6 (72%), Folate (67%)	Impaired energy production	Fatigue
	Vitamin E (86%)	Lower levels of vitamin E to protect cell membrane	Lipid peroxidation
	Phenolics, phytosterols	Lower availability of antioxidants	Lower levels or phenolics and phytosterols reduce the availability of dietary antioxidants. This puts greater stress on the body's manufactured antioxidant known as gluthathione. This can then affect the inflammatory process.[33]
	Fibre (resistant starch, fructans, cellulose, hemocellulose, arabinoxylans, lignin, germ, cellulose, B vitamins and vitamin E)	Lowered fecal bulking Poor glycaemic regulation Insufficient prebiotic supply such as inulin that contributes to the health of the small intestine while restricting growth of Escherichia coli, salmonella and listeria, and increased absorption of minerals (i.e. calcium)[34]	Increased susceptibility to constipation Increased risk of hyper/hypoglycemia Possible impact on gut flora prebiotic supply

If damage to fat occurs to the cell membrane, the process is called lipid peroxidation. Research shows that children with autism tend to have more tiny 'fires' (oxidation), resulting in a higher level of lipid peroxidation. When a child's diet is low in vitamin E, lipid peroxidation is more likely to occur.[35] The brain is particularly vulnerable to lipid (fatty) damage due to its high (60%) fat content. If the fatty membranes that insulate the brain cell enhance processing speed for thoughts, any damage to this fatty layer may affect cognitive function, such as thinking and reasoning.[36]

Vitamin E is not the only antioxidant present in wholegrains – a whole range of tiny plant nutrients is present. Plant sterols, little fatty-like substances, also offer antioxidant protection, and antioxidant support plays a role in reducing inflammation. Children with autism appear to have higher levels of inflammation. Much like the little 'fires', inflammation can continue over time. In health, inflammation has a temporary purpose, usually to respond to infections or injuries. But when inflammation becomes chronic, it can affect many functions of the body, including the brain. Although the science in this area is still in its infancy, research has shown that a pro-inflammatory state may affect our ability to process information. For example, many instruments in an orchestra don't necessarily mean good melody and harmony – all the rhythms and notes need to come together for a clear musical tune to be played. Inflammation is one way that synchronization can affect our brain's orchestra and slow down processing.

Children with autism produce higher levels of immune-activating proteins known as cytokines that can play a role in driving inflammation. These can be switched on and off according to need. When we produce too many of these, or they do not switch off after time, we can have longer-term inflammation. John Welsh and fellow researchers wrote about the slower processing in the brain of children with autism, and that this slower effect can affect language and communication.[37] Therefore, our aim is to use an anti-inflammatory diet to reduce the overall levels of inflammation in the body. An anti-inflammatory diet allows plant nutrients, such as plant sterols and phenols, to switch off pro-inflammatory proteins when they are no longer needed.

The question we need to ask is, what is the principle we need to follow when choosing starchy carbohydrates? Based on the importance of all these different nutrients as well as maintaining healthy gut flora, the obvious answer would be wholefoods in a more natural state. This means wholegrain rice, potatoes in their skins such as new potatoes, cereals such as oats or wholegrains without additional sugars added. In theory this is sound, but in practice, this can be a challenge. In Part II we look at ways we can begin to introduce more natural wholefood choices.

Fruits and Vegetables

The pattern of fruit and vegetable intake varies considerably between children. Some eat plenty of fruit and drank lots of fruit juice, while others avoided fruit altogether. Bananas seem to be a popular choice, followed by apples, grapes, raisins, berries and pears.

Fruits and vegetables are supernourishing. Fruits contain higher levels of sugars than vegetables, including glucose, fructose and sucrose. Fructose is a single fruit sugar, and sucrose is made up of two sugars: fructose and glucose. All these sugars are present in varying amounts in fruits and vegetables. Some fruits, such as bananas, have high levels of sugar, whilst others, such as blueberries, contain lower sugar levels – bananas contain three times more sugars than equal amounts of blueberries.

Any processing of fruit concentrates the sugars. Examples of processing include fruit juice or dried fruit. A portion of fresh grapes (50g) contains 7.7g of sugar; dried fruit, such as a box of raisins (28.3g) contains 19.6g of sugar; and a glass (250ml) of grape juice contains 29g of sugars. Both dried fruit and fruit juice significantly increase sugar intake, so a principle with choosing fruit options is to choose fresh fruit where possible. Lower sugar fruits can be chosen where a child cannot tolerate fruit well. Reducing fruit juice intake or diluting juice with water or avoiding fruit juices for a time are options if a child has issues around yeast or bacterial overgrowth, and symptoms such as bloating or diarrhoea. Replacing some fruit intake with more vegetables is another alternative for children who do not tolerate fruit well.

We need to acknowledge that many children do not like vegetables, especially green vegetables. Issues with colour, taste and texture might make any vegetable aversion worse. In clinic we notice that very few vegetables are eaten, although most of the time children whose parents follow a traditional Asian, African or Middle Eastern diet tend to eat more vegetables. Carrots and broccoli are commonly reported, along with tomatoes and sweetcorn, and peas, although not defined as vegetables, are included in the vegetable list. The research supports this pattern, showing fewer portions of vegetables, salads and fruits being eaten by children with autism.[38]

It is difficult to over-exaggerate the importance of vegetables in the diet. Table 2.4 shows the beneficial effects of eating a diet rich in green leafy vegetables, thus demonstrating the possible benefits that are lost in a diet lacking green leafy vegetables. These nutrients play many roles, including cell protection and DNA repair, healthy gut flora, reducing inflammation and supporting detoxification.

Table 2.4: Benefits of eating a diet rich in green leafy vegetables

Nutrient	Benefits	Benefical action
Glucosinolates	Switch off inflammation from bacterial lipopolysaccharide	Anti-inflammatory
	Anti-infective (e.g. inhibiting H. pylori) Anti-viral activity	Immune supportive
Folate	Improved methylation	Reduction in hyperactivity
Lycopene Zeaxanthin Beta-carotene Astaxanthin	Anti-oxidant	Protection against oxidative damage[39]

If there is a family of vegetables that is well known for its health benefits, it is the *cruciferous family*, containing kale, watercress, rocket, lamb's lettuce and spring cabbage, to name a few. These vegetables are well-known for their sugar–sulphur nutrients known as glucosinolates, bitter in taste, but powerful in their health-boosting activity. One of these activities is protecting deoxyribonucleic acid (DNA). DNA is the genetic material in the cell, a genetic instruction book telling the body what it needs to produce in every circumstance. Its method of communication is protein. Protein instructions tell our body to make hormones and enzymes – they are immune messengers and much more. Not all instructions are communicated (expressed). Communication or expression occurs when the diet and environment talk to the genes and influence what it says. For example, broccoli has tiny ingredients that tell the genes to communicate in proteins the message, 'produce more phase 2 detoxification enzymes'.[40] DNA is constantly unravelling and recoiling, and during this process, things can get stuck to it. This can damage the DNA and affect its function, which will affect the clarity of its instructions. When there is miscommunication, there is always the possibility of compromised function.

Green leafy vegetables also help the immune system. Many children with autism have suppressed immune function, so any dietary support, such as the anti-viral and anti-bacterial activity of vegetables, will be supportive to the body.

We cannot mention green leafy vegetables without discussing their relation to the folate family of nutrients. Folate is the natural dietary form of folic acid. Rather than having one or a few shapes like the supplemental form, the dietary form has hundreds of different shapes and sizes. Some children with autism have a genetic variation for an enzyme known as methylenetetrahydrofolate reductase (MTHFR 677T/TT). The genetic variation (MTHFR C677T/TT) is for a gene that codes for an enzyme called methylenetetrahydrofolate reductase (MTHFR). This is a long name for a little protein enzyme that is part of a cycle known as the methylation cycle. This allows the body to switch genes on and off, to make new fat units for the cell membrane, repair brain and gut cells, regulate the neurotransmitter function, and activate nutrients and much more. In these individuals, gene MTHFR C677T/TT variation results in the enzyme being less active.[41]

Some scientists recommend a higher folate intake for these individuals, 660µg rather than 400µg.[42] Eating foods rich in folate can negate some of the natural effects of having this MTHFR C677T gene variation, and help the methylation cycle to work more efficiently.

Much folate is lost by cooking or canning vegetables – higher levels of folate are present in fresh, uncooked produce. Fresh green leafy vegetables such as rocket and romaine, butterhead, rosso and oakleaf lettuce can supply rich sources of folate that can be eaten raw or added to food once cooked (as they easily wilt).

If children have an aversion to green vegetables, you can always try white versions of the brassicas such as cauliflower or turnip. Colourful vegetables are also encouraged – the more variety, colour and range, the wider the range of protective plant nutrient function.

A principle when choosing vegetables is to choose those that are grown locally and organically, to maximize nutrient content, and then to choose plenty of green leafy vegetables, if tolerated. Spinach, due to oxalate levels, is better replaced with lower oxalate options, or rotated. Colourful vegetables should also be eaten. If a child has an aversion or problem with one vegetable, find an alternative vegetable to replace it. In Part II there are a number of methods to increase vegetable content.

Proteins

In our study dietary patterns for protein show that some children avoid protein and others ate high quantities of meat and very little carbohydrate. This variation in protein intake is also seen in the research. Dietary sources of proteins include meat, fish, beans, nuts and vegetarian meat-style alternatives such as Quorn® or textured vegetarian protein.

Breakfast

The typical pattern of protein intake at breakfast includes omelettes, or fried, scrambled or poached eggs. Some families following special diets such as the specific carbohydrate or GAPS diet (Gut and Psychology Syndrome), eat larger quantities of eggs. Meat-based sausages and bacon are also a popular choice. Sometimes vegetarian sausages or baked beans are eaten. Yoghurt could also be considered to be a protein-rich food, as a small pot of 125g contains 7.1g of protein, the same amount of protein as in an egg. Cow, goat or soya milk yoghurts are frequently eaten, and less frequently, coconut milk yoghurt. As many children can have an issue with both cow's milk and soya milk yoghurt, there are a few homemade yoghurt-like recipes in Chapter 4 that can easily be prepared at home.

Lunch/Evening Meal

Protein sources at lunch/evening meals include meats such as chicken, mince (ground meat), steak, burgers and sausages, and highly processed meats and fish such as chicken nuggets, ham, chicken, turkey slices or fish fingers. Beans and lentils are sometimes also added to stews or soups. Nuts are eaten on their own or in cereal bars. The research supports what we see in clinic, with increased intake of processed proteins such as chicken nuggets and hot dogs.[43]

Table 2.5 shows examples of different types of processed proteins and eggs, with the types of nutrients lost/ingredients added or negative effects and intolerances. It also shows the possible effect on nutrients.

Table 2.5: Examples of different types of processed proteins and eggs

Typical protein choices	Nutrients lost in processed proteins/ ingredients added that have a negative effect/ intolerances	Functional impact	Symptoms
Ham Bacon Sausages Turkey slices	Preservatives added to ham, bacon and sausages. Sodium nitrate is added and can be converted into nitrites by the gut bacteria.	Elevated nitrites and nitrates are observed in autism, leading to oxidative stress and inflammation. Behavioural changes are observed in animals exposed to sodium nitrate.	Distractibility, headaches, hyperactivity.
Chicken nuggets Fish fingers	Can be deep-fried, creating increased levels of trans fats.	Trans fats can replace essential fatty acids in the brain cells.	Trans fats can adversely affect cognitive function.
Fish	Can contain contaminants such as methylmercury. Larger fish have a greater concentration (i.e. marlin – 10–20 times more methylmercury per kg than salmon and trout, tuna – 4–5 times more than salmon).	Inorganic and organic mercury have been associated with pro-inflammatory reactions.	Muscle pain, sensitivity to sound, hand-flapping, problems with comprehension.
Eggs (some people can tolerate eggs in some forms and not others, e.g. boiled or eggs in baked goods)	Egg allergy is one of the top eight food-related allergies.	Allergic response symptoms.	Constipation, eczema, additional symptoms associated with egg allergy or sensitivity.[44]

Table 2.5 also shows some of the challenges faced by children with autism when eating processed meats. Processed meats usually contain preservatives and nitrates. Nitrates can be naturally occurring, but some children with autism find them difficult to process, and respond with hyperactivity. It is preferable to replace processed meats such as ham and bacon with less processed organic or grass-fed meats. We talk more about meat choices later, in Chapter 3.

When thinking about protein, especially animal protein, we need to consider the types of fat it contains and the cooking process. Trans or damaged fats are often produced in the process of frying or synthesized as a cheaper solid fat option to add to foods. If we eat this type of fat, the body will try to incorporate it into the cell membrane. Trans fats have been linked to greater levels of aggression and irritability, so we want to reduce or eliminate them from the diet.

Proteins from fish also need to be thought about as they can contain various levels of toxins such as methylmercury. Mercury has often been associated with certain behaviours, and symptoms seen in autism.

Proteins such as eggs, fish, nuts and soya are amongst the top eight allergens. Some groups of children we see have multiple food sensitivities or allergies. This can be quite a challenge, especially when the children are already on quite a restricted diet. So it is necessary to look at the diet carefully to ensure there is adequate protein intake.

There are a number of ways of calculating protein intake. First is using dietary recommended intakes, such as the recommended daily allowance for protein. There is ongoing debate about optimum levels of protein intake, but the RDA can be used as a guideline. Table 2.6 shows the RDA of protein for various age groups, with examples of daily portions of protein that would make up that RDA.

Table 2.6: Recommended daily allowance for protein

Age (years)	Protein RDA (g/day)	Examples of daily portions (g/day) for one day's intake for corresponding daily RDA
1–3	13	2 tbsp lentils (24.6g) = 2.2g 1 pot CO YO™ yoghurt (125ml) = 2.9g 2 tsp pumpkin seed butter = 2.9g Quinoa flakes (40g) = 5.4g
4–8	19	Small portion of lamb mince (ground meat) stew (60g) = 14.6g Oat porridge (40g) = 5g
9–13	34	1 chicken breast (90g) = 29g 12 almonds (12g) = 2.5g Chickpeas (40g) = 2.9g
14–18	52 (male), 46 (female)	1 salmon steak (100g) = 23g 1 egg = 7.1g 3 tbsp green beans (60g) = 1g Small portion of millet (100g) = 3.5g Small baked sweet potato (98g) = 1.6g 1 portion of soba (buckwheat) noodles = 5.8g 1 pot soya yoghurt = 4.7g (+ extra 6g for male)

Fats

Dairy-free margarines, butter, ghee (clarified), coconut oil and other oils such as sunflower or olive oil are commonly reported in the food diaries. Some of the parents also report regular intake of shop-bought gluten-free products. Trans fats are present in higher levels in gluten-free products. This includes gluten-free pastries, cakes, biscuits and crackers. Eating a gluten-free diet, where most foods are shop-bought, may expose children with autism to higher levels of trans fats.

Ghee or clarified butter is also sometimes eaten to a greater extent in diets such as the GAPS diet. Ghee is another potential source of trans fats. Trans fats are considered to be three times more likely to promote fat deposits in the artery compared to saturated fats, and are linked to systematic inflammation.[45] Table 2.7 show examples of how poor quality fats can affect the body's function, and the effects that can occur as a result of eating certain types of fats.

Table 2.7: Examples of poor quality fats

Typical food choices	Functional impact	Symptoms
Poor quality fat Gluten-free products (processed cakes and biscuits), which tend to have higher levels of hydrogenated/trans fats Fats from animal products like meats or hard cheeses Margarine Fried foods such as potato chips	Increased damage to fats. Vitamin E destroyed when frying oil and reheating oils. Increased lipid peroxidation.[46] Trans fat interferes with production of DHA, a very long chain omega-3 fatty acid that is thought to be protective against aggression, altering energy production, and causing oxidative stress and inflammatory effects.	Effects on cell membrane fluidity and inflammation Associations between atopic conditions (asthma, eczema, hay fever) and trans fats Decreased insulin sensitivity and trans fats Aggression and irritability[47]

Fats from meats are also a major source of fat intake. Sausages can contain up to 60 per cent fat. High fat content combined with high sugar is not a good combination. Sugar can create reactions in the blood that lead to damaged fats. Protecting fats as they travel through the blood is important. This protection comes from antioxidant-rich foods such as vegetables and fruit. So, if a diet is higher in fat, it should also be higher in fruits and/or vegetables and low in sugars, to enhance overall protection.

When choosing fats in the diet, the general principles are to choose fats in as natural a state as possible. Plant fats, when eaten naturally, are usually packed with plant sterols and other protective nutrients. High-fat plant foods include avocado, nuts, seeds and coconut. Examples of a more natural processing of fats would include soaking high-fat plant foods such as seeds or nuts, and then making salad or vegetable dressings, creams and 'yoghurts'. This way, the fat will be easier to digest as the seed has been soaked and blended. And cooking methods such as frying, roasting and baking can damage the structure of the fat, to some degree. So cooking foods at a lower temperature is an option, or using water-based methods of cooking, such as steaming.

Dairy

When we review the pattern of dairy intake, children can be divided into several groups – those who already eat a gluten- and casein-free diet, those who are just casein-free, those who limit the amount of dairy they eat or who eat an average amount of dairy, and those who have excessive cravings for dairy products, drinking pints of milk daily.

Full fat cow's milk, soya, rice milk or coconut milk are commonly used. Soy is the most commonly used dairy alternative, with soya yoghurt often replacing dairy yoghurt. The good thing about soy is that it probably makes the most comparable non-dairy food product. The challenge is, however, that it is also a top allergen. Children with cow's milk allergy often have problems with soy as well. Sensitization to pollen, such as birch tree pollen, can also cross-react in the body, making the child also sensitive to a food such as soy. After soy, rice milk is most commonly used. Dairy-free cheese alternatives are rarely eaten. The literature also shows that many children with autism tend to have a lower intake of dairy overall.[48]

The main challenge of excluding a wholefood group from the diet is the loss of nutrients that the food group would naturally supply. In the case of dairy, this would be mostly protein and calcium. Although some plant-based milks such as almond milk have naturally occurring calcium, most dairy-free milks have to be fortified in order to deliver equal amounts of calcium per serving as cow's milk. This means that parents have to check to see if the dairy-free milk is fortified. Fortified soya, rice, oats and almond milk show comparable levels of calcium to dairy milk, unlike hemp milk, which contains one-third of the calcium found in cow's milk. One cup of milk (250ml) or a portion of milk on cereal (135ml) will not be sufficient to supply the recommended daily calcium requirements. Children aged 1–3 have a calcium requirement of 500mg daily; those aged 4–8, 800mg daily; and those aged 9–18, up to 1300mg daily.

We have to remember that removing dairy from the diet not only removes milk, but other dairy sources of calcium such as yoghurt (commonly eaten by children) and cheese. Often dairy-free alternatives are not used to replace these items, resulting in a greater overall loss in calcium from the diet.

It is important that calcium is replaced if dairy is removed from the diet, either with calcium-rich foods or using supplemental sources. Most often it is a challenge to meet the calcium requirements using diet alone. This can be an issue, as children with autism can have a reduction in bone cortical thickness on the casein-free diet compared to those who had minimally restricted or unrestricted diets.[49]

Table 2.8: Examples of calcium-rich foods

Food source	Portion size	Calcium content (mg)
Sardines	4–5 sardines (100g)	500
Tofu	½ cup (125g)	438
Hemp milk	1 cup (250ml)	300
Coconut milk (e.g. Koko®)	1 cup (250ml)	300
Whole milk (cow's)	1 cup (250ml)	295
Goat's milk	1 cup (250ml)	250
Almond milk	1 cup (250ml)	300
Sesame seeds	1 tbsp	74
Flaxseed/linseed	1 tbsp	90
Kale	1 cup (67g)	87
Rocket	1 cup (30g)	48
Watercress	1 cup (30g)	51
Yoghurt (cow's), Greek	1 small pot (125g)	158
Yoghurt (coconut, e.g. CO YO™)	1 small pot (125g)	9.9
Yoghurt (soya)	1 small pot (125g)	14.9

Source: Nutritics Professional Dietary Analysis Software (2014).

Dairy exclusion can result in a significant reduction of calcium intake, and dietary intake of calcium alone may not be sufficient to meet the recommended calcium intake. When considering dairy exclusion, even as a trial, it is important to discuss with a dietician, nutritionist or doctor how calcium can be replaced.

Drinks

Patterns of soft drink intake include lots of orange juice, apple juice, smoothies and blackcurrant juice drinks. Many drinks contain additives or natural flavourings that promote hyperactivity in some children, as well as high sugar levels. On average there is about 20g of sugar per 100g in cordials or fruit juices. Lower sugar drinks often use artificial sweeteners. Table 2.9 shows some examples of fruit juices and cordials, including low-sugar options.

Fruit juices contain little or no fibre. This speeds the entry of sugar into the circulation, and can lead to blood sugar spiking. There is also the issue of how sugars can affect the overall carbohydrate digesting capacity. It would make sense that if a child has issues with fructose digestion or general digestion, reducing fruit juices can be a good place to start. Of course if the child is eating no fruits or vegetables, it is important to think how any lost nutrients will be replaced. The fluid intake itself can be replaced by drinking water or fresh homemade juices. Cutting out smoothies and juices can be a major challenge, so subtly adding in extra water may be one of the ways to begin. We look at various drink recipes later, in Chapter 8.

Table 2.9: Nutritional value of fruit juices and drinks

Juices and drinks	Quantity (ml)	Energy (Kcal)	Carb.	Sugars
Apple juice, unsweetened	200	76	19.8	19.8
Fruit drink, Ribena® (all flavours ready to drink)	200	108	26	19.6
Orange juice, from concentrate	200	74	18	18
Robinsons® Fruit Shoots, no added sugar	200	10	1.6	1.6
Tropicana® orange juice	200	94	20	20
Innocent® smoothie (strawberries and bananas)	200	108	24	21

Source: Nutritics Professional Dietary Analysis Software (2014).

Snacking

Many children tend to graze on snacks throughout the day. Snacks generally consist of rice cakes, biscuits (i.e. jam tarts, digestive biscuits, chocolate biscuits) and gluten-free biscuits, cheese, processed cheese and various types of yoghurts. Table 2.10 shows the calorie, carbohydrate, protein, fat, fibre and sugar content for a selection of snack portions. High fat or high-protein snacks help with better regulation of blood sugar to avoid blood sugar dips. Sugary snacks tend to make the blood sugar rise quite sharply. Combining a snack like a rice cake with a protein choice such as sunflower seed butter helps to prevent any sharp sugar rises.

Children who snack continually often seem to have persistent bloating and flatulence. Continual snacking on highly processed carbohydrates is likely to increase the risk of small intestine bacterial overgrowth, due to constant intake of foods that may then take longer to process due to constant eating. A principle for snacking would be to have the snacks at regular times rather than continually since this would allow the digestive system to know when to respond, and gives it at least a little break for restoration and recovery.

Table 2.10: Nutritional value of snacks

Food name	Portion	Energy (Kcal)	Carb.	Protein	Fat	Fibre	Sugars
Cheese, English Cheddar	1 slice	92	0	5.6	7.7	0	0
Chocolate chip cookies	3	128	17.6	1.6	6.2	0	8.5
Chocolate chip cookies, gluten-free	3	121	16.4	1.2	6	0.1	9.2
Jam tarts, shop-bought	2	130	22	1.1	5	0	12.2
Rice cakes	3	89	19.5	2	0.9	1.4	0.2
Yoghurt, Müller Fruit Corner®, all flavours	1 pot	158	22	5.7	5.7	0.8	22

Source: Nutritics Professional Dietary Analysis Software (2014).

Working Together

We have looked at the various dietary patterns seen in clinic for children who first attend, and notice that many nutrients are lost due to highly processed dietary choices. With this in mind, our aim should be to try to raise nutrient intake.

Whilst we could ask questions about foods rich in specific nutrients, such as foods rich in iron or B vitamins, we know that nutrients never appear in isolation. They are concentrated in foods and work together synergistically.

Many nutrients working together underline the importance of a varied wholefood diet, making the need to eat wholefoods much more than the intake of single vitamins, minerals or plant nutrients, and more than a variation in fatty acids and proteins. Diversity brings greater stability. Supernourishing food, then, gives the body the chance to have a comprehensive spectrum of protective nutrient cover.

Energy production is a good example of nutrient synergy, and is essential for every function of the body. Let's take understanding and communication, for example. Although many factors can affect understanding and communication, clues from specific illnesses can help us understand how these can be affected. Patients who develop viral or bacterial encephalitis (swelling of the brain) can experience loss of speech.[50] Mitochondrial disease or dysfunction can also affect comprehension and speech. Any problem with the way the mitochondria work (the energy factories of the body) or redirection of energy can effect understanding and communication. We have all experienced energy lapses when the body re-directs its energy from thinking and communication to fighting an infection. The flu is a good example of this. Tiredness and low blood sugar are additional examples. A high degree of coordination and synchronization in the brain is needed for comprehension. Different areas of the brain come together and synchronize their rhythms, allowing us to make sense of the world. It is a bit like playing a musical tune in an orchestra. Insufficient energy production can affect the rhythms of the brain, and thus affect the harmony or clarity of any musical tune played (an analogy for comprehension or speech). So anything that might affect these rhythms can also impact and slow down processing speed, thus affecting comprehension and speech.

Synergy: Nutrients Working to Make Energy

The diagram below shows a mitochondria, where most of the body's energy is made. It shows an example of nutrients working together. Energy production uses a super enzyme called pyruvate dehydrogenase that powers the conversion of carbohydrates and proteins to enter the energy cycle. Pyruvate dehydrogenase uses many B vitamins such as B1, B2, B3 and B5, as well as lipoic acid, a sulphur-containing fatty nutrient. B vitamins are lost when grains are refined, but refined grains still need their carbohydrates processed to make energy. So we need to borrow B vitamins from elsewhere. This might mean that another cycle that needs B vitamins may not work as well.

Carbohydrate, fat or protein enter the energy cycle and then continue to need B vitamins, minerals such as iron, magnesium and manganese, and amino acids such as cysteine. Some nutrients play 'keystone' roles. Magnesium is an example of this. It is required at most of the steps of energy production, so if it is low, symptoms of fatigue may be seen.

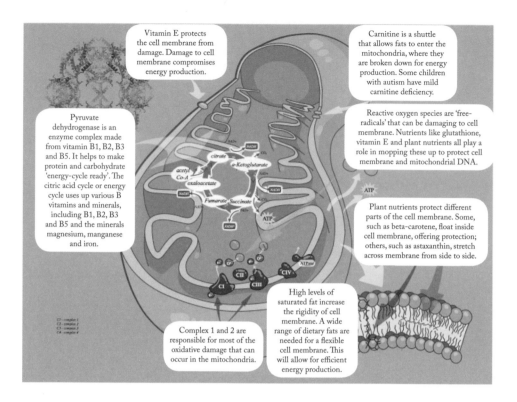

Eighty per cent of the energy needed for the cell is made in the membrane of the mitochondria. This means we need lots of healthy flexible membrane to pump around the energy. Flexibility requires diversity, a range of dietary fats, fats of different length, shape and structure, and omega-3 fats such as docosahexanoic acid (DHA), eicosapentanoic acid (EPA), alpha-linoleic acid, gamma-linolenic acid, healthy monounsaturated, polyunsaturated and saturated fats. Too many fat strands of saturated fats, and the cell membrane becomes more solid, compromising energy production.

But it is not just eating the right fats that is important. Special assembly of the fats so they are 'mitochondria membrane-ready' requires assembly by another nutrient-hungry cycle called the methylation cycle. This cycle has many functions, including switching genes on and off, making new fat units for the cell membrane, repairing brain and gut cells, activating nutrients and much more. Again, specific B vitamins including B12 are required for this cycle as well as dietary folate. Low levels of folate or B12 can then affect production of healthy cell membrane building blocks.

The mitochondria uses up 85 per cent of the cells' oxygen during energy production. The oxygen use needs to be carefully controlled. Part of the oxygen management system requires nutrients such as manganese, copper and zinc. It also needs good amounts of glutathione, a protein-based antioxidant generated by the body. For a number of reasons, glutathione is often lower in children with autism, so plant nutrients provide a back-up system to preserve the antioxidant glutathione. This again reminds us that we need rich sources of wholefood plant nutrition to protect this oxygen-rich environment to slow any tipping towards membrane damage.

Dietary sources of antioxidants are in a class of their own, varying in shape and size – these influence how they submerge into the cell membrane. Beta-carotene is a powerful antioxidant present in carrot sticks, papaya-based smoothies and green juices. Beta-carotene can lie on its back in the cell membrane. Another family member also found in some orange fruits and vegetables is astaxanthin, which can stretch from one side of the cell membrane to another. This allows for more diverse cell membrane protection, thus taking the pressure off glutathione.

Curcumin from the root spice turmeric is also protective. It can be added to juices, soups or curry, and particularly likes to protect the energy-pumping complexes. Damage to these complexes can result in increased oxidative stress, and reduced antioxidant supplies, and over time, can lead to inflammation.

Finally, it is not only nutrients for the mitochondrial membrane or for manufacturing its building blocks that need consideration. We need to think about the activity of mitochondria as it moves through the cell to meet energy demands. Impeded movement can affect the way energy is produced. Soft scaffolding in the forms of tiny strips of protein known as actin allow the mitochondria to keep afloat in the cell, and shift to areas where more energy is needed (such as when the brain needs extra energy during learning). To keep this system working well we can't have debris floating around and interacting with the scaffolding. We need to detoxify substances that can get into the cell from the environment, such as heavy metals. Detoxification is quite a heavy user of nutrients, and we need this function to help to remove unwanted stuff from cells and the body. So again, we see the importance of diet and nutrients working synergistically in multiple pathways to support energy production.[51]

In this simplified explanation of energy production, we see how nutrients working together reinforce the need for a whole spectrum of nutrients that can only be obtained from a wholefood diet. We also see that many children with autism may choose highly processed foods, resulting in removal of some of these nutrients. Naturally we need to think about increasing supernourishing foods in the diet. The recipes in Part II aim to offer options so this can be done.

In Chapter 3 we look at the food groups with the aim of highlighting some of the challenges faced in a group of children who sometimes have a high degree of sensitivity to various foods.

3 Poor Digestion, Sensitivities and Allergies

We have looked at the highly processed diet often eaten by children with autism. These highly processed food choices frequently have many of their nutrients removed, resulting in lower overall nutrient intake. Our concern is that over time, this can negatively influence the body's efficiency. We used the illustration of energy production to show the need of a wholefood diet and nutrient synergy to help the body to function.

We are now going to review the food groups, looking at benefits and challenges within each group. These challenges are not exclusive to autism, but rather to food sensitivities and allergies, poor digestion, imbalance in gut flora and increased gastrointestinal permeability.

Increased gastrointestinal permeability happens when the little threads that hold the gut cells together get frayed and break down, allowing the passage of incompletely digested foods, bacteria and other substances from the gut to the circulation.[52]

From this review, we hope that we can suggest principles, as well as precautions, that are relevant for children with autism, with our overarching goal to encourage supernourishment.

Five Food Groups

Five food groups are normally recommended as part of a balanced diet. In the UK there is a picture diagram, known as the *eatwell plate*, where the food groups are divided into carbohydrates, fruits and vegetables, proteins, dairy and dairy alternatives, and oils and sugars.

In the US this is called *MyPlate* and is divided into four groups, with a fifth group as a cup on the side of the plate containing dairy. The *MyPlate* food guide is divided into grains, protein, fruits and vegetables, with bigger portions for grains and vegetables. Unlike the UK's plate, the US plate does not have a portion to illustrate fats or sugary foods.

The illustration below shows an example of a healthy plate, with a high intake of wholegrain, plant-based and minimally processed foods.

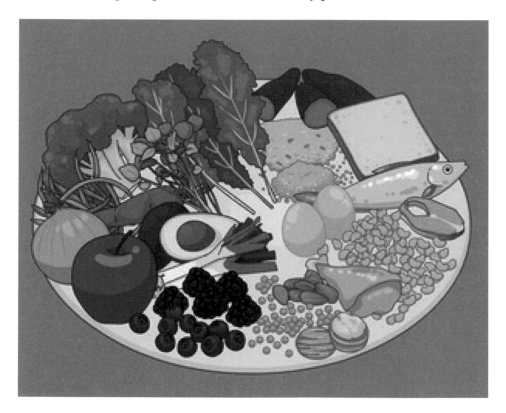

Picture diagrams are helpful for visualizing food groups representing a balanced diet, but they do not really help us understand which food within a group is a healthier choice. For example, which is healthier – frozen fruit or tinned fruit?

The food plates are also limited as they are designed for the general population. Their recommendations are relevant to large groups of people within the population, but need modifying for people with complex needs. Such needs are often seen in children with autism who sometimes present with malabsorption issues, chronic infections, gastroesophageal reflux disease (GERD) or symptoms of irritable bowel syndrome (IBS).

As a parent or carer, it can be difficult to know how to modify a child's diet. So the continual reminder is to see a clinician who is experienced and knowledgeable about food, so they can guide appropriately. This is especially true when working with children who are growing and already have multiple issues including 'picky' eating, health problems and restricted diets.

In the following section the food groups are divided up slightly differently into fruits and vegetables, carbohydrates, dairy, proteins and fats.

Fruits and Vegetables

Fruits and vegetables are the most nutrient-dense food per calorie. This means that they are generally low in fat and carbohydrates, and higher in water content. In their natural state, fruits and vegetables are also high in fibre. Apart from fruit, nuts/seeds and grains, no other food contains fibre.

We have already spoken a little bit about fibre and blood sugar balance, and fibre as a bulking agent, but fibre is so much more functional than that. Just as one example, we can look at beta-glucan. This is found in grains (e.g. oats), mushrooms and seaweed. The fibre-like substance helps to stimulate the immune system, reduce oxidative stress (the little 'fires'), protect the cell membrane and preserve glutathione levels.[53]

Fruits and vegetables are also a source of sugars and short chain carbohydrates. These include glucose, fructose and sucrose. They also contain slightly longer chains of sugars (3–10 units). These are usually good for you, and are known as prebiotics, and act as food to keep gut bugs healthy. Oligosaccharides (meaning many sugars) and galactooligosaccharides (meaning milk sugars, although not just found in milk) are two examples of probiotics.

Probiotics and Prebiotics

Probiotics can be defined as live bacteria or yeasts that, when taken in sufficient quantity, can offer health benefits to the person taking them. Foods such as kimchi and sauerkraut contain good levels of probiotics.

A prebiotic is a type of fermentable fibre that promotes the growth of the probiotic. Foods rich in prebiotics include onions, leeks, garlic, legumes, Jerusalem artichokes and chicory root.

Fruits and vegetables also contain thousands of plant nutrients. These have many health-promoting features, including switching genes on and off. In autism the body is usually in a more 'revved-up' state, driven by higher levels of oxidative stress.[54] Plant nutrients can play a role in switching the genes on and off more efficiently, even when body is revving.

Plant nutrients have so many additional benefits that it would be impossible to list them all, therefore only some of the protective effects are listed below. This list relates to benefits in cancer prevention, although these are obviously not only relevant for one health issue – they are transferable benefits. We can look at the benefit of detoxification again. Nutrients from fruit and vegetables enhance the detoxification process. Low levels of fruit and vegetables in the diet are likely to compromise the body's ability to detoxify well.[55] It would make sense that if fruits and vegetables provide protective and functional effects in the body, reduced fruits and vegetables in the diet could then result in lower levels of protection and function. Most of the research looking at populations, diet and disease supports this idea.

Examples of potential mechanisms of action of dietary phytochemicals for cancer prevention are:

- antioxidant activity
- DNA repair
- regulation of cell and system communication (signal transduction)
- enhanced detoxification
- anti-inflammatory
- enhancement of immune function and surveillance
- anti-bacterial
- anti-viral effect.[56]

Even though fruits and vegetables can be so beneficial, some people have problems processing them. Part of the reason for this was outlined earlier – food sensitivities, poor digestive function, problems with small intestine bacterial overgrowth and gut microbiome imbalances, nutrient deficiencies and problems with processing and eliminating substances from the body. We could umbrella all the issues that people face when eating fruits and vegetables under gut microbiome imbalance, poor digestion, and food sensitivities or allergies. The first challenge, then, is one of digestion and absorption, and that is seen in the way the body processes sugars and short-chain carbohydrates.

Short-Chain Carbohydrates

Carbohydrates vary in length, from 1 unit of sugar to thousands of units. Little carbohydrates are about 1–60 sugar units long. These are broken down by enzymes (disaccharides) that are embedded along the micro-fingers that line the small intestine. Any irritation to the gut, excess mucus production, small intestine bacterial overgrowth and lower levels of disaccharide enzymes and transporters can lead to poor digestion and absorption. If you are not digesting well, you might not be getting enough nutrients, and can experience symptoms such as bloating, flatulence, diarrhoea and offensive stools. Eating habits such as gulping food or grazing can worsen any symptoms already associated with poor digestion.

We have already looked at the way small short-chain carbohydrates can draw water into the intestines and promote diarrhoea, and how flatulence is promoted by overgrown bacteria producing excess gas, but we have not mentioned the knock-on effect of poor carbohydrate digestion. If carbohydrates are not being digested well, and there is an increase in small intestine bacterial overgrowth, it is not only carbohydrates that will be affected. The environment that poor carbohydrate digestion creates will catch both fats and protein in the cross-fire. It may be that a child already has compromised protein digestion due to low stomach acid, or low levels of protein-digesting enzymes, but this can be made worse if there is also a fermenting slow bowel movement. If poor protein digestion is present, symptoms are often experienced, including offensive or smelly stools, undigested foods in the stools and fat in the stools (oily film on water, lighter coloured stools).

The presence of the symptoms of bloating, flatulence and diarrhoea are common in children with autism, and are also seen in IBS. A diet called the FODMAP diet looks at the type of carbohydrates eaten, and is often recommended for IBS-like symptoms in certain sensitive individuals.

FODMAP DIET

So what is the FODMAP diet? FODMAP stands for fermentable, oligo-, di-, monosaccharides and polyols (FODMAPs). In short, these carbohydrates can be rapidly broken down by bacteria in the bowel and ferment easily. Sugars are joined together in strings of various lengths. Oligosaccharides usually have fewer than ten units of sugars. Disaccharides, double sugars, have two units. Monosaccharides have one sugar unit. Polyols have sugar alcohols including sorbitol, mannitol and xylitol.

FRUCTOSE

Fructose is a single sugar found in fruits, vegetables, honey and high-fructose corn syrup, and is combined with glucose in sucrose. Some children with autism do better on a low-fructose diet. In this case, choosing a fruit that contains lower levels of fructose may be an option, or choosing more vegetables, as vegetables are naturally lower in fructose. Table 3.1 shows the carbohydrate, fibre, sugars, glucose, fructose and sucrose levels of various fruit.

Sweeteners such as honey and agave syrup have very high levels of fructose compared to those found in sweeteners such as molasses, and most cane sugars including coconut palm sugar.

One word of warning about fruit sugars is that some lower-fructose fruits may be higher in sucrose. Bananas are good examples of this, as they are lower in fructose but higher in sucrose. Looking at total fruit sugars in a fruit is helpful in assessing overall sugar content.

High total sugar fruits, fruit juices and dried fruit can be problematic for children who have challenges with yeast/bacterial overgrowth and yeast/bacterial flares. They can also be a problem due to the high glycaemic index (GI) levels, promoting quick release of sugars into the blood. Pairing fruits with nuts is a good way to lower the overall GI release from fruit. If there are nut or seed allergies, beans can be used instead.

Glycaemic Index (GI)

The glycaemic index (GI) is a ranking system that shows the overall response of blood sugar levels to foods eaten. Higher GI foods raise sugar levels more quickly than lower GI foods.

Table 3.1: Nutritional value of a variety of fruits and vegetables

Food name	Qty (g)	Carb.	Fibre	Sugars	Glucose	Fructose	Sucrose
Goji berries, dried	100	68	8	37	8.6	8.7	0
Grapes, average	100	15.4	0.8	15.4	7.6	7.8	0.1
Pears, raw, average portion	100	10	2.8	10	2.3	7.1	0.7
Apples, eating, raw, average portion	100	11.8	2.1	11.8	1.7	6.2	3.9
Bananas, weighed without skin	100	23	3.1	21	4.8	5	11.1
Kiwi fruit	100	10.6	2.3	10.3	4.6	4.3	1.3
Bilberries or blueberries	100	6.9	2.5	6.9	3.3	3.3	0.4
Mangoes, raw, ripe	100	14.1	2.9	13.8	0.7	3	10.1
Strawberries, raw	100	6	2	6	2.6	3	0.3
Papaya, raw, flesh only	100	8.8	2.3	8.8	2.8	2.8	3.1
Raspberries, raw	100	4.6	6.7	4.6	1.9	2.4	0.2
Grapefruit, raw	100	6.8	1.6	6.8	2.1	2.3	2.4
Melon, cantaloupe	100	4.2	0.9	4.2	1.8	2.2	0.1
Plums, raw, average portion	100	8.8	2.3	8.8	4.3	2	2.5
Carrots, raw	100	7.9	2.6	7.4	2.3	1.9	3.2
Lemons, whole, without pips	100	3.2	1.1	3.2	1.4	1.4	0.4
Nectarines	100	9	2	9	1.3	1.3	6.3
Cranberries	100	3.4	3.8	3.4	2.2	1.2	0
Green beans/ French beans, raw	100	3.2	2.7	2.3	0.8	1.1	0.4
Curly kale, raw	100	1.4	3.7	1.3	0.6	0.6	0.1
Sugar-snap peas, raw	100	5	0	3.7	2.4	0.4	0.9
Lime juice, fresh, weighed whole	100	0.7	0	0.7	0.3	0.3	0.1
Beetroot, raw	100	7.6	2.3	7	0.2	0.1	6.7

FRUCTANS

We all are aware that cabbages and legumes can be associated with flatulence, and fructans are one of the reasons why. These small chains of fructose–fructose bonds should break down in the large intestine. However, when there is constipation, small intestine bacterial overgrowth, excessive mucus production or low levels of disaccharides, these can be easily fermented. Foods that contain fructans include chickpeas, wheat and rye and various fruits, vegetables and legumes. I have included examples of fructan-rich foods and low-fructan alternatives in Table 3.2 below. For more information on these, read Dr Sue Shepherd and Dr Peter Gibson's book, *The Complete Low-FODMAP Diet*.[57]

Table 3.2: Fructan-rich foods and lower fructan alternatives

Food group	Fructan-rich foods	Lower fructan alternatives	
Fruits	Nectarines Peaches Persimmon Watermelon	Most other fruits	
Vegetables	Globe and Jerusalem artichokes Beetroot Cabbage Garlic Leeks	Avocado Bok choy Broccoli Cauliflower Chives Green beans Lettuce	Pumpkin Spring onions (scallions) Squash Swedes Sweet potatoes
Cereals, grains and starches	Wheat- and rye-based products	Buckwheat Millet Oats	Quinoa Rice Tapioca
Legumes	Chickpeas Legumes (including borlotti, haricot (navy), pinto, lima, butter, adzuki, soy, mung, broad) Lentils	Regular tea and coffee Herbal tea	
Nuts/seeds	Pistachios	Almonds Linseeds	Sunflower seeds
Fibre supplements	Inulin and fructo-oligosaccharides (FOS)		

POLYOLS

Polyols are sugars with a little alcohol chain attached. They can be helpful for some children and unhelpful for others. Cherries and cauliflower can work wonders to help speed bowel movement in the more constipated child, whereas diarrhoea can occur in those with more loose stools. Polyols are present in apples, watermelon and pears, and again, can be associated with bloating.

Table 3.3: Polyol-rich and low-polyol foods

Food	Polyol-rich foods	Low-polyol foods
Fruits	Apples, pears, blackberries, cherries, apricots, nectarines, peaches, plums, prunes and watermelon	Bananas, blueberries, cranberries, grapefruit, grapes, honeydew melon, kiwi, lemons, limes, mandarins, mangoes, oranges, passion fruit, papaya, pineapple, raspberries, rhubarb, strawberries
Vegetables	Avocado Cauliflower Mushrooms Mange tout (snow peas)	Everything apart from the polyol-rich foods listed in the first column
Diet, sugar-free or low-carb foods	Gum, mint, lollies, polyols such as mannitol or xylitol	Gum sweetened with sucrose
Additives	Sorbitol (E420), mannitol (E421), maltitol (E965), xylitol (E967)	Aspartame, saccharine, stevia

This brief review of small-chain carbohydrates makes us realize that diet can be very complicated for people with digestive issues. In practice, I have seen that it is not only about specific foods that are eaten, but the diet as a whole. The more the diet is harmonized with principles that support healthy digestion, the more the sensitive gut can tolerate variation. This can take time, though, needing skilled professionals to design nutritionally adequate dietary choices for the growing child.

The next section looks at how in addition to poor digestion, an imbalanced gut microbiome can lead to overproduction of substances such as phenols and salicylates that overwhelm the processing pathways.

Phenols and Salicylates

Phenols and salicylates are the plant nutrients that give the colour, flavour and benefits to foods such as fruits, vegetables, grains and nuts (see Chapter 2 for a discussion on the benefits of these nutrients).

Like everything we eat, drink or are exposed to in our environment, plant nutrients need to be used by the body, and then broken down and eliminated. Plant nutrients are broken down through various processing pathways. If these pathways are overwhelmed, the nutrients or other similar substances will stay in circulation for longer, giving rise to unwanted symptoms.

One of the ways that the processing systems can become overwhelmed is when there is an imbalance in the gut microbiota. This complex community that lives in the gut is constantly producing different substances that can help or cause problems in the body. It is also partly responsible for maintaining a healthy gut lining, and building mucosal scaffolding to maintain the surface of the gut in good health.[58] When the community become imbalanced through antibiotics, anti-fungals, a high intake of processed sugars or highly processed carbohydrates, poor digestion, high stress levels, or even certain medications such as proton pump inhibitors (medication that lowers stomach acid pH), there is an overgrowth of specific strains of bacteria. Examples of this reported in autism include Ruminococcus, Clostridium species (including C. histolyticum, C. tetani, C. perfringens and C. bolteae), Desulfovibrio and Sutterella. Repeated use of antibiotics can create an environment that is more favourable for one or more toxin-producing bacteria, increasing their 'population'.[59]

The result of increased 'toxin-producing' bacteria is greater production of substances to be broken down and eliminated via processing pathways. We use enzymes to break things down in the body. Some of the enzymes the body uses need sulphate to work properly. The challenge is that some children with autism lack sufficient sulphate in their blood. Some suggest that this is partly due to a higher excretion of sulphate through the urine, or reduced nutrients needed for sulphate production;[60] others suggest explanations such as an increase in the bacteria Desulfovibrio, a sulphate-loving bacteria whose levels are associated with increased severity in autism. So low sulphate levels affect the processing capacity of certain pathways.

One of the pathways that low sulphate affects is the pathway that processes phenol, a ring-like shape that is in foods, places in nature and in our environment. We can normally break phenols down, but sometimes our ability to do this is compromised by bacterial overgrowth, due to over-production of phenol shapes, overwhelming the breakdown pathway. Clostridia produces para-Cresol, the phenol shape that is also present in the environment in rainwater, disinfectants, artificial flavours, foods such as tomato ketchup, bacon, smoked foods, cheese, butter and asparagus.

Imagine a combination of phenols coming in from the environment, food, bacterial overgrowth and then on top of this, your processing power is working slower than it should be. What happens? Something has to give. In my clinical experience, and from speaking to other clinicians and parents, some of the symptoms associated with 'phenol sensitivity' include hyperactivity, emotional extremes, dark circles under the eyes, red face and ears, headache, difficulty falling asleep at night, night waking, tiredness and lethargy.

It would also appear that children with phenol sensitivity have different tolerance thresholds. They can tolerate smaller amounts of phenol-rich foods, but if they eat too many, the balance is tipped. Factors such as bacterial overgrowth may also influence the level of 'sensitivity'. Looking at improving the gut microbiota seems to help some children tolerate phenol-rich foods more readily, whilst others benefit from rotation between low- and high-phenol foods.

Phenol levels in fruit and vegetables vary considerably depending on where the food is grown or if it is sun-ripened. Table 3.4 lists a variety of fruits and vegetables. There are no recommendations for levels of phenols. High-phenol foods are usually nutrient-packed and include darker fruit and vegetables, chocolate, dried fruits, spices and herbs.

Salicylates are another phenol shape. These are present in vegetables, fruit and spices, as well as medicines (such as aspirin), flavourings and perfumes. The degree of salicylate sensitivity varies between people. Again, it can be quite a serious issue in some children, and needs to be evaluated by someone who has experience dealing with salicylate sensitivity. Symptoms of salicylate sensitivity include bed-wetting, dermatitis, ear infections, fatigue, headaches, hypoglycemia, a persistent cough, lethargy, runny nose, sleep disorders, agitation and hyperactivity.[62]

When phenol or salicylate-rich foods are replaced with lower-phenol/salicylate foods in children with 'phenol sensitivity', parents observe improvements, although it is worth pointing out that the symptoms that have been associated with phenol sensitivity may be driven by other factors. Phenol sensitivity is not a problem for all children with autism. Because of the nutritional benefits of phenol-rich foods, careful evaluation of the child's symptoms and diet is necessary under the supervision of an experienced clinician.

Table 3.4: Polyphenol levels of certain fruits and vegetables[61]

Fruits	Total polyphenols (mg/100g) (Folin assay)	Vegetables	Total polyphenols (mg/100g) (Folin assay)
Watermelon	1.84	Celery	13
Passion fruit	57	Cucumber	21
Papaya	58	Fennel	28
Honeydew melon	59	Courgette (zucchini)	30
Lemon	60	Celeriac	59
Pear	108	Leek	62
Grape (green)	122	Green lettuce	66
Pineapple	148	Sauerkraut	67
Banana	155	Asparagus	75
Grapefruit	163	Onion (golden)	76
Kiwi	180	Cauliflower	82
Grape (black)	185	Pumpkin	86
Apple	202	Cabbage	89
Blueberry	223	Napa cabbage	116
Orange	279	Rocket	136
American cranberry	315	Avocado	152
Plum	410	Beetroot	164
Date	488	Kale	177
Blackberry	569	Sweet pepper	181
Blackcurrant	821	Bok choy	193
Figs (dried)	960	Broccoli	198
Raisins (grape)	1065	Spinach	249
Prunes	1195	Dandelion leaves	386

Oxalates

Oxalates are tiny salts present in varying amounts in plant foods. Children with autism are thought to have three times more oxalate in their plasma than that of neurotypical children.[63] In the paper titled 'A potential pathogenic role of oxalate in autism', Konstantynowicz and colleagues suggest that there could be a link between sub-clinical intestinal inflammation and increased absorption and availability of oxalate. There is also a question of whether imbalanced gut flora plays a role. Anti-fungal programmes seem to lower the excretion of oxalates. Certain bacteria such as Oxalobacter formigenes are also thought to be helpful, although they may be destroyed by antibiotics. However, both the bacteria Lactobacillus acidophilus and Bifidobacterium lactis are thought to help with oxalate breakdown.

Certain nutrients can be helpful for some children, such as calcium or magnesium citrate. These citrates can bind to the salts and decrease absorption. In addition, vitamin B6 helps the enzyme that breaks down oxalate alanine-glyoxylate aminotransferase (AGT).

Macronutrients such as excessive fats also increase the availability of oxalates in the diet because fats absorb the calcium that would normally bind to the oxalate. Taurine supplementation may also be helpful as it helps to stimulate bile production, and thus helps with fat digestion. Calcium citrate can also reduce oxalate absorption.[64]

Food Intolerances and Biogenic Amines

Phenols and salicylates are not the only tiny substances that can create unwelcome symptoms in children. Biogenic amines are a biologically active compound including chemicals such as histamine, brain transmitters such as dopamine, and mono or single amines known as tyramine, which have been associated with headaches.

We may be familiar with the effects of histamine, with reddening of the skin and sometimes itchiness and swelling after a cut or insect bite. This is a normal reaction. But in some people, these reactions are more pronounced or last for longer than they should. People who have problems with amines such as histamine can experience allergic-like symptoms (e.g. runny nose, racing heartbeat, low blood pressure, itching, diarrhoea, oedema on the eyelids, flushing, headaches, migraines, asthma, shortness of breath, or fatigue following meals). Histamine and tyramine occur naturally in the body and also in food, or can be generated in the gut. If your body produces too much histamine and/or you have problems breaking it down, you can develop sensitivity to histamine, which is also known as histamine intolerance. This is when a person experiences a greater severity of symptoms associated with increased amounts of histamine ingested.[65]

Foods containing histamine may trigger various symptoms. Foods that are dried and fermented, including products such as dried anchovies, fish sauce, fermented vegetables (e.g. sauerkraut and kimchi), cheese, fermented sausages, beer and preserved meats, as well as fermented soy products (e.g. Miso or soy sauce), can trigger this type of reaction.

In a healthy person, histamine from the diet is broken down using enzymes known as amine oxidases (e.g. diamine oxidase). These enzymes can be affected by genetic variation, nutrient insufficiency, GI problems such as gastritis, bacterial flares, food allergy, eczema, hypertension or vitamin B6 deficiency. Fermented vegetables such as sauerkraut also tend to have quite a high level of histamine as well as other amines, and some children do not react well when eating these types of foods. If a food intolerance reaction that is driven by bacterial overgrowth occurs, rebalancing the gut flora can help to reduce some of the symptoms experienced.

Allergies

Finally, we need to consider allergies. An allergy to fruits and vegetables is becoming increasingly common. This is partly due to increasing cross-reactions between foods and airborne substances like pollen. Children often become sensitized to inhalant allergens first, and then later develop allergies to fruit and vegetables. Examples of cross reactions include ragweed pollen cross-reacting with banana, cucumber, melon and courgette (zucchini), and birch pollen cross-reacting with peaches, apricots, cherries and plums.

Some children also have contact dermatitis where they will have a reaction between their skin and the pulp of a fruit. Lemons, tangerines, limes, oranges and grapefruit can provoke this type of reaction.

Allergies to one fruit or vegetable can increase the chances of reacting to another; for example, melon increases the risk of a response to avocado and banana. Latex also cross-reacts with banana, avocado and coconut. Medical examination and various tests can be conducted to evaluate possible allergies.

Fruits and vegetables are an indispensable part of a healthy diet. We know that children with autism often have basic challenges in eating enough fruit and vegetables due to picky eating. From Chapter 2 we can see that over time this can lead to nutrient deficiencies. In this chapter we have highlighted some of the challenges that children with autism who have specific food sensitivities or allergies can face when eating certain fruits and vegetables. The great thing about fruits and vegetables is that there is so much variety, and replacing nutrients through varying the fruits and vegetables eaten can be done effectively. However, the key point is that every child is different. And we cannot assume because a dietary change worked for one child that it will work for another. Equally, without the guidance of a skilled professional, there is a chance that the diet can become nutritionally inadequate.

Carbohydrates

The second food group is the starchy carbohydrates. These take up a third of the *eatwell plate*. This group is made up of tuber vegetables such as potatoes, sweet potatoes, yams and grain or pseudo-grains. They contain high levels of carbohydrate, between 15 and 90g per 100g. The nutritional density and health benefits of carbohydrates can vary considerably, however, depending on the level of food processing.

Nutritional density, GI, fibre levels, food allergies or intolerances, carbohydrate content, fructan content and method of processing are all issues that may need to be considered when choosing starchy carbohydrates.

Nutritional density varies between different choices of carbohydrates, as discussed in Chapter 2. Nutrients are reduced when fibre is removed, and over-processing reduces phytonutrients, vitamins, minerals and oils.

Even if wheat-containing bread or cereals are made with processed grains, where fibre and bran is removed, the law requires manufacturers to fortify them with certain vitamins. This is not true for gluten-free products, although some gluten-free manufacturers do fortify their bread with fibre and B vitamins. It is worth checking if the gluten-free bread or cereals are fortified, as grains and grain-like foods are a major source of B vitamins.

In Table 3.5, the gluten-free bread is fortified. Natural high fibre levels are present in both the wholemeal bread and the pumpernickel bread. Crispy rice cereal has a much lower level of fibre. Eating breakfast cereals with low fibre levels can impact bowel movement, so it is worth considering how to increase fibre at breakfast time, especially for children who are quite resistant to change. In Chapter 4 we look at some ideas of how to add fibre to cereals to increase the nutritional density at the beginning, when first transitioning the diet to more healthy options.

When a grain is ground into flour or puffed, as in rice cakes, the GI increases. Wholemeal bread will have a higher GI (24) compared to pumpernickel bread (14.4) made from wholegrain. Biona® makes a range of gluten-free breads that are similar to pumpernickel bread, but some children may not like the texture or taste. Alternatively, you could try making your own gluten-free bread. Try the Sunflower Butter Bread recipe in Chapter 5.

Wholegrains have a lower GI than rice cakes or crispy rice cereal. So wholegrain millet porridge is preferable to Rice Krispies® for breakfast, due to the slower release of sugars. Lower GI breakfasts are preferable because breakfast sets up the regulation of insulin and blood sugar for the day. In this way, a more balanced blood sugar can positively affect the immune system, help to influence inflammation, and hopefully have a positive knock-on effect on brain dynamics, helping to reduce melt-downs and poor concentration.

Table 3.5: Nutritional content of breads and cereal products

Food product	Qty (g)	Carb.	Fibre	Zinc	Vit. B1	Vit. B2	Vit. B3	Folate
Bread roll, fibre, gluten-free, fortified Glutafin	35	15.1	2.1	0.6	0.1	0	2.3	20
Bread, pumpernickel	35	15.8	2.3	0.5	0.1	0.1	1.1	33
Brown rice, basmati, boiled	35	9.7	0.2	0.1	0	0	0.6	1.9
Chapattis made with fat	35	16.9	1.9	0.4	0.1	0	1.2	5.3
Rice cakes	35	25	1.8	0.6	0	0	2.1	6
Crispy rice cereal	35	29	0.5	0.4	0.5	0.6	6.8	70
White bread, average	35	17.3	0.8	0.2	0.1	0	1.2	10.2
Wholemeal bread, average	35	14.7	2.5	0.6	0.1	0	2.1	14

Because carbohydrate content between different food products varies quite considerably, such as the difference between 35g of new potatoes boiled in their skin, which contains 5.4g, compared with one packet of a potato crisps 'grab bag' containing 18.7g of carbohydrate, it would be preferable not to overload the digesting capacity of the gut by eating carbohydrates from highly processed carbohydrate-rich sources. In the case of potato, it would mean choosing boiled new potatoes and not potato crisps. This isn't to say that potato crisps can't be eaten, but why not rotate them with vegetable crisps or vegetable snacks such as carrot sticks?

This also highlights the wisdom in introducing a larger amount of homemade baked products. And if shop-bought gluten-free products are used, then think about the options that can be easily made to replace some of these.[66] This leads us on to the topic of gluten.

Gluten

The starchy carbohydrate group also contains grains that can contain gluten. Gluten is a protein storage unit for grain and grain-like seeds. The protein storage unit is known as a prolamin. These prolamins or proteins are present in all grains, including gluten-free grains.

Table 3.6: Grains and prolamins

Grain	Prolamin	% of protein in grain
Wheat	Gliadin	69
Rye	Secalinin	30–50
Oats	Avenin	16
Barley	Hordein	46–52
Corn	Zein	40
Rice	Orzenin	55
Millet	Pennisetin	5
Sorghum	Kafirin	52

Table 3.6 shows grains with the levels of protein storage (prolamin's) in grain/ pseudo grain and percentage of protein in the grain. You can see that certain grains have a greater amount of prolamins (proteins) than others. The less protein the grain contains, the easier it should be to digest. Soaking grains helps to begin the unravelling process, making the protein easier to digest.

There are many different explanations about why gluten is thought to be an issue for some children with autism. One of these suggests that gluten-derived peptides (little protein chains) trigger an immune response, resulting in an excessive gastrointestinal inflammation. Researchers found that children with autism had a stronger pro-inflammatory response to food proteins from gluten, casein and soy, compared to non-autistic controls.[67]

There is also debate about whether children with autism experience a greater incidence of coeliac disease, with some studies suggesting a link and others not. I wonder if it is only a sub-group of children who might be at a greater risk leading to some of these conflicting results. Some studies show an increased risk of markers associated with coeliac disease without a corresponding positive biopsy. Others suggest non-coeliac gluten sensitivity as a possibility.[68]

Fructans

Finally we meet fructans again. The main source of fructans are wheat- and rye-containing products such as bread, pasta and cereals. Wholegrain flour contains higher levels of fructans than white flour, and might explain why some people can tolerate white flour better than wholegrain. Bloating and digestive discomfort are some of the symptoms experienced when you can't tolerate fructans.

The way we process grains can make a big difference in helping to make the nutrients more available. Like all plant seeds, grains, nuts, seeds and beans all contain substances that can have an effect on mineral absorption. In order to maximize absorption from wholegrains, we need to activate the enzyme phytase to break down the phytates present in the grains and seeds. This is done by soaking the grain, nut or bean before cooking. Breads that use sprouted grains are examples of this. Lactic acid-producing bacteria often used in a sour dough starter also help this process.

Try soaking cereals overnight. Soaking rice before cooking speeds the cooking process, lowers phytates and makes the rice more digestible. Soaking rice in warm water produces anxiety-calming substances such as gamma-amino butyric acid (GABA).[69] Finally, soaking can also reduce oxalates. Table 3.7 shows grains and grain-like seeds and soy with oxalate in mg levels per 100g.

Table 3.7: Grains and grain-like seeds and soy and their oxalate levels[70]

Grain/grain-like food	Oxalate (mg/100g)
Buckwheat	269
Soy	183
Barley	67
Cornmeal	56
Dark rye	54
Semolina	51
Unbleached white flour	48
Brown rice	37

Principles in choosing breads would always include a process that encourages longer fermentation of the bread, like sour dough bread. Where possible, grains should be soaked or sprouted, and eaten by slower chewing or having them blended.

Dairy and Dairy Alternatives

A dairy product is a food produced from the milk of a mammal. This can include milk and food products made from cows, goats, sheep and even camels. Common dairy products include cheese, cream, yoghurt, ice cream, cheesecakes, and many other foods. Milk, cheese and yoghurt are probably the most commonly used dairy products in children with autism.

In the *eatwell* and *MyPlate*, a portion of dairy is included. This is because dairy products are rich in calcium. The recommended daily intake of calcium is quite high, making it difficult to achieve daily calcium requirements when dairy is omitted from the diet. As a result of this, the use of fortified foods or supplementation is often needed.

Table 3.8: Body systems affected by cow's milk allergy and symptoms produced

Systems	Symptoms
Skin	Raised itchy rash (urticaria) Angioedema (swollen lips) Inflammation of the skin (dermatitis)
GI	Abdominal pain Diarrhoea Oral itching Nausea Gastroenteritis Eosinophilic esophagitis Colic Constipation Gastroesophageal reflux
Respiratory	Runny nose Red eyes Sneezing Blocked nose Worsening of symptoms with asthma Breathing difficulty

Having an allergy is probably one of the more frequent reasons why dairy is excluded from the diet. Non-IgE mediated cow's milk protein allergy can gives rise to symptoms of diarrhoea, constipation, alternating diarrhoea, bloating and abdominal cramping. There is usually a history of colic and vomiting in early infancy, and diarrhoea and loose stools in older children.

There also seems to be cross-reactivity with a milk allergy (affecting 2–3% of children). Some children with a milk allergy have an increased sensitivity to eggs, soy, goat's milk and sometimes beef protein.

Dairy-free alternatives like soy can also produce similar symptoms to a cow's milk allergy (see Table 3.8), including enterocolitis (inflammation of the digestive tract).[71]

Lactose Intolerance

Bloating is a very common symptom seen in autism, and is associated with poor digestion. This might mean that the sugar in the milk rather than the protein is a potential source of the bloating. Lactose intolerance is associated with symptoms of bloating, flatulence, diarrhoea, stomach cramps and rumbling, and nausea. Lower levels of the milk-digesting enzyme lactase can increase the range or degree of symptoms.

Not all dairy products contain equal amounts of lactose. This is why some people can tolerate cheese but not milk. In Table 3.9 below, examples of varying lactose levels in different portions of dairy products are given.

Butter and cheese have negligible levels, compared to the high levels in whole milk. People with lactose intolerance can sometimes tolerate foods with low lactose levels, while others do better on lactose-free dairy products. Lactose intolerance can be worse after viral infections, while probiotics can improve the tolerance of dairy products in some people.[72]

Table 3.9: Lactose levels in different portions of dairy products

Food name	Measure	Lactose (g)
Butter	1 tsp	0
Cheese, English Cheddar	1 slice	0
Cream, fresh, double	1 tbsp	0.3
Ice cream, dairy, premium	Average portion	1.6
Evaporated milk, whole	1 tbsp	2.1
Yoghurt, whole milk, fruit	1 small pot	5
Whole milk, pasteurized, average	On cereal	6.2

Dairy-free products are naturally casein- and lactose-free. Many children with autism use dairy-free alternatives. The biggest challenge when replacing dairy is that there is a significant loss of calcium intake in the diet. Many dairy-free milks have been fortified with calcium to contain similar amounts per ml to cow's milk. Table 3.10 compares some of the pros and cons of different dairy-free choices.

Table 3.10: Dairy-free milk alternatives

Groups	Dairy-free milk alternatives	Cons	Pros
Grains	Rice Oats Millet Quinoa Teff	Contain starchy carbohydrates. Can have high GI. Rice can have higher levels of arsenic (best to rotate grains).	Easy to access Fortified Alternative to soy and nuts Appropriate for low oxalate diet
Legumes	Soya Pea	Soya allergy (some cross reaction with peanuts). Peas can cause problems with amines.	Easy to access in many different forms. Have shown protective effects for DNA adducts (an adduct is a foreign substance that can get stuck to the DNA affecting its ability to instruct the cell correctly)
Nuts	Almond Cashew	Almonds are high in oxalates. Very low levels of almond used (2%). Maltodextrin and other sugars and preservatives or thickeners are used. Can cause an allergy.	If made at home, offer whole fats Readily available
Seeds	Sunflower Pumpkin Coconut	Moderate oxalates. Coconut can be a FODMAP problem. Sunflower and pumpkin are not easy to access.	Coconut is easy to access Pleasant flavour

Added sweeteners/thickeners: agave syrup, maltodextrin, guar gum (can be difficult to digest)
Environmental: BPA (Bispherol A, a plasticizer that can affect hormone regulation) lining of aluminium cartons and tins

Calcium is constantly needed for remodelling and growing bones. Children with autism have been found to have high markers for inflammation. It is believed that this inflammation can affect bone health in children with GI conditions such as Crohn's disease.[73]

Vitamin D is also important for calcium absorption. Vitamin D intake, and vitamin D receptor genetic variation, can also influence calcium levels. Low stomach acid can also affect calcium absorption, making supplementing calcium citrate or malate a better option as they are more water-soluble. Bran, fibre and phytates can all lower calcium uptake. Efficiency of calcium absorption is better when supplements are given in divided doses. Table 3.11 shows the recommended dietary allowances for children between the ages of 0 and 18 (see Chapter 2 for a list of potential sources of calcium). It is important to ensure that calcium is replaced either through the diet or supplementation. Medical or licensed health professional advice is needed to ensure that the diet is nutritionally adequate.

Table 3.11: Recommended dietary allowances of calcium

Age	Calcium (mg)	Vitamin D (Qg)
0–6 months	210	5
6–12 months	270	5
1–3 years	500	5
4–8 years	800	5
9–18 years	1300	5

Proteins

Proteins are vital for every function in the body. In Chapter 2, we learned that children with autism can eat too much or too little protein. They sometimes have problems with protein due to textures or chewing difficulties. Others may experience bloating after eating foods like beans.

Animal proteins include meat, poultry, fish; dairy products such as cheese or yoghurt; and also eggs. Plant proteins include beans and pulses, grains, nuts and seeds. Meat substitutes such as Quorn®, soya or wheat-based protein are other sources of protein. The major difference between animal and plant protein is the amino acid composition, variation in fibre (there is no fibre in meat), and differences in types of fats and phytonutrient composition.

When considering some of the issues that children with autism face in relation to protein as a food group, we have to think about the source of protein, how the protein is processed, how it is cooked, bacterial levels and possible contaminants. In addition to this, we need to consider the tiny ingredients or additives that a child may be sensitive to. Protein-rich foods are usually quite allergenic due to their high protein content. Fish, crustaceans, eggs, tree nuts, peanuts, soya and milk are all protein-rich foods, and are seven of the eight top allergens.

Finally, we have to think about what constitutes adequate protein intake, as protein is needed for every function of the body and is important in growth and repair. But first, we should consider the difference between meats based on the way the animal is reared and fed.

Grass Versus Grain-Fed Cattle

Not all meat is of equal quality. When meat from grass- and grain-fed animals is compared, grass-fed animals tend to produce meat that is richer in nutrients and that contains a healthier ratio of fats.

Animals fed grass have higher levels of beta-carotene, vitamin E and glutathione compared to grain-fed cattle. Grass-fed meat also costs twice as much money to produce as non-grass-fed meat. The specific types of saturated fats associated with grain-fed animals have a more negative cholesterol profile. Grass-fed cattle have significantly higher levels of omega-3 fatty acids.[74]

Although grass-fed meat is pricier, if the portion size of the meat is reduced in recipes, replacing some of the meat protein with plant protein, this not only allows for a higher quality meat to be used, but also, due to the plant nutrient-rich protein, this enhances the overall nutrition value of the protein. Adding pulses to stews, and beans to burgers, patties or sausages, is a good way of doing this.

Processing Proteins

Making your own sausages and burgers using lean meat and adding in vegetables or plant protein is preferable, although not always possible. So, looking at ingredients such as fillers and additives, as well as overall fat levels, is quite important – even tiny amounts of certain ingredients can set off a very sensitive child.

Sausages, cured meats, smoked foods and cheese are preserved using various processes. Nitrates and nitrites are mineral salts that can be used as preservatives. Once in the body, they can be converted into nitrosamines, a chemical that may be associated with cognitive and neuropsychiatric impairment.[75] As an alternative to these preservatives, celery salt is sometimes added to sausages or meats. Garlic, lemon and citrus products are thought to help to reduce nitrate levels.

A final consideration is how protein has been processed in terms of adding other ingredients such as breadcrumbs or batter, and whether it is deep-fried, or if the protein has been salted or smoked. Replacing fish fingers, chicken nuggets, hot dogs, bacon and chicken slices with their more natural alternatives is preferable. Our major aim is to choose proteins that are nutrient-rich and minimally processed.

Cooking Methods

Like any other food, the cooking method will influence the health value. Chargrilling, frying or cooking at high temperatures promotes the forming of chemicals in the muscle of the meat known as heterocyclic aromatic hydrocarbons. These chemicals can stick to DNA and affect its function. Although I do not promote frying or cooking foods at very high temperatures, the reality is that sometimes food is cooked in this way. The use of the cruciferous vegetable family can be quite helpful to support removal of these products through a process called phase 2 detoxification. Supersprouts such as broccoli sprouts can powerfully induce phase 2 enzymes.[76]

Juicing greens is another way of bringing in nutrients to support detoxification pathways. One study looked at the effects of drinking 100ml of wheat grass juice daily. Continuous reduction of Bisphenol A (a plasticizer) took place over the two weeks.[77] Additionally, low oxalate vegetables such as bok choy (pak choi), kale, cauliflower, kohlrabi, watercress and broccoli can all be used to support detoxification.

Reducing or avoiding grilling and barbecuing, turning meat over more frequently, and removing charred portions of meat are all ways of reducing the presence of these substances in the diet. Alternative methods of cooking include poaching, stewing, braising and steaming, or even frying at lower temperatures.[78]

Bacteria in Meat

It is worth considering some of the research looking at bacterial levels in meat. Bacteria like Clostridium difficile was frequently found in 50 per cent of beef and 42.9 per cent of pork in meats in the US. Clostridia perfringens was present in 66 per cent of fresh chicken and 67 per cent of frozen chicken.[79] Cooking at high temperatures can reduce bacterial count, but some are concerned that heating kicks in the spore-forming process.[80] Oils with anti-microbial properties such as cumin and clove oil can be added to meat to reduce levels of Clostridia. Rosemary oil is known to reduce C. difficile. Adding the oils once the meat is cooked helps to reduce growth of C. perfringens. Recipes for herb, cumin and clove oils, to add to meats once cooked, are given in Chapter 6.

Fish and Toxins

Eating fish has become quite a controversial topic due to its beneficial fatty acids and concern about the various ocean pollutants. These include metals such as arsenic (inorganic) or mercury (methylmercury), organochlorine and organophosphate pesticides, herbicides, polycyclic aromatic hydrocarbons, polychlorinated biphenyls and dioxins (a by-product of herbicide production). As you can imagine, it would be difficult to get lists of fish showing the levels of each of these substances, as they vary according to fish size, fat stores, wild versus farmed fish, temperature of water, location, how old the fish is, if it is a filter feeder like shellfish or a predator like tuna, and how healthy the fish is in terms of its ability to detoxify.

The US Food and Drug Administration site[81] lists mercury levels in commercial fish and shellfish from 1999–2010. In Table 3.12 I have selected fish from that list to give some idea of the concentration of mercury, parts per million (PPM), in different varieties of fish.

It is worth mentioning that concentrations of other pollutants will vary between species, but the general rule is to choose smaller, younger and 'happy' fish (such as wild fish). Smaller portions and a variety of species are recommended, together with cooking foods alongside the fish that support detoxification processes.[82] Fish such as anchovies, salmon, sardines and pollock are some of the higher EPA/DHA (eicosapentaenoic acid and docosahexaenoic acid) varieties for higher intake of the omega-3 fatty acids with lower levels of mercury concentration (see Table 3.12).

Table 3.12: Average mercury concentration for various fish and seafood[83]

Species	Average (mean) mercury concentration (PPM)
Scallop	0.003
Salmon, canned	0.008
Sardine	0.013
Tilapia	0.013
Anchovies	0.017
Salmon, fresh/frozen	0.022
Pollock	0.031
Mackerel, Atlantic	0.050
Haddock, Atlantic	0.055
Butterfish	0.058
Trout, freshwater	0.071
Hake	0.079
Whitefish	0.089
Lobster, North American	0.107
Carp	0.110
Cod	0.111
Perch	0.121
Skate	0.137
Tuna, fresh/frozen – skipjack	0.144
Bass, saltwater, black, striped	0.152
Snapper	0.166
Halibut	0.241
Tuna, fresh/frozen	0.391
Grouper, all species	0.448
Marlin	0.485
Tuna, fresh/frozen – bigeye	0.689
King mackerel	0.730
Shark	0.979
Swordfish	0.995

Source: US Food and Drug Administration (2014).

Plant Proteins

Plant proteins are nutrient-packed. Examples of protein-rich plant sources are nuts, seeds and beans. Their amino acid composition varies between plant proteins and animal proteins. Plant proteins tend to have lower levels of essential amino acids and overall protein. Methionine (an amino acid) is called a limiting amino acid in beans, as there are lower levels of methionine compared to animal proteins. Grains, in contrast, have higher levels of methionine, hence the suggestion that grains and beans should be combined to improve the amino acid ratios.

Plant proteins have higher levels of phytonutrients than animal proteins. They also contain fibre where plant proteins contains none. These extra plant nutrients offer protective benefits to any fats that plants contain. Both nuts and seeds are also rich sources of fats, so these nutrients offer protective effects. Plant-rich protein foods can also pass on some of their benefits to the fats found in animal proteins if they are combined. Research is looking at how plant and animal protein can be combined to promote greater health benefits. One of the lines of investigation is the use of plant fibres. These are being added to sausages or burgers to increase overall health value. Nuts or beans can also be added for some of the reasons listed above.

Beans are known for many of their health-promoting properties. One of the key benefits is their low GI. They are also rich in prebiotics (feeding gut bugs) and fibre, and have been associated with decreased risk for diabetes and heart disease. This suggests that they help to support both improved blood sugar regulation and healthier blood flow and blood vessels. Any improvement in blood sugar regulation or blood flow will have a knock-on positive effect on inflammation. Galactooligosaccharides are an example of a prebiotic, and can play a role in inducing detoxifying enzymes, stimulating immune function, regulating lipid and hormone metabolism, as well as other health effects.[84] They are also rich in B complex vitamins and minerals.[85]

Not everyone can tolerate beans, and there are a number of reasons for this. The prebiotic fibres promote fermentation, and so can lead to increased gas production, bloating and flatulence. They also contain other substances such as lectins. These are a complex sugar-binding protein that can irritate a sensitive gut lining. If beans are not prepared properly, they also have higher levels of anti-nutrient substances like trypsin inhibitors, lectins and phytates. Kidney beans have higher levels of lectins compared to white beans, lentils or green peas or beans.

Trypsin (protein enzyme) can inhibit protein digestion, but it can also have a positive effect on protecting DNA.

Processing both beans and nuts plays an important part in helping to make these proteins easier to digest. Soaking is a major method for helping to improve digestibility. Soaking beans in boiling water helps to reduce both lectins and oligosaccharides.[86] The longer the soaking time, and the higher the soaking temperatures, the more the lectin levels are reduced, and the better the oligosaccharides start to break down. Recommendations suggest soaking beans and pulses overnight as a minimum, although soaking for 48 hours is preferable. Soaking beans helps to break down and reduce the fibres present, and it also breaks down some of the digestive enzyme inhibitors, as does cooking them at a high temperature. You can also choose pulses without skins, such as red lentils, split peas or urid lentils (without skins).

Phenols

As with fruit and vegetables, some nuts and seeds also have higher levels of phenols. Table 3.13 gives examples of different levels in a selection of nuts, seeds and beans.

Table 3.13: Examples of high-phenol and low-phenol nuts, seeds and beans[87]

Food	Higher phenols	Lower phenols
Nuts and seeds	Almonds (287mg)	Macadamia (126mg)
	Brazils (244mg)	Pine nuts (58mg)
	Cashews (233mg)	Walnuts (28.50mg)
	Hazelnuts (687mg)	
	Pecans (1816mg)	
	Pistachios (1420mg)	
Beans	Adzuki (8970mg)	Peas (119mg)

Soaking and sprouting can be helpful in reducing phenols. Soaking beans for 12 hours significantly reduces polyphenols by 27 per cent. Sprouting beans prior to cooking can reduce phenols by over 50 per cent. Pressure cooking is also an effective way of reducing phenols.[88]

Oxalates

Oxalates, as discussed in the Fruits and Vegetables section above, are also present in nuts and beans. Many children do not have oxalate issues, but some do. Table 3.14 is a guide to oxalate levels in some nuts and beans. Oxalate levels can also be reduced by soaking.

Table 3.14: Levels of oxalates in a selection of nuts, seeds and beans[89]

Nuts	Oxalate (mg/100g)	Beans	Oxalate (mg/100g)
Almonds, roasted	469	Black	72
Cashews, roasted	262	Soy	56
Hazelnuts, raw	222	Pinto	27
Pine nuts, raw	198	Aduki	25
Peanuts, roasted	140	Red kidney	16
Walnuts, raw	74	Chickpeas	9
Pecans, raw	64	Mung	8
Pistachio nuts (roasted)	49	Lentils	8
Macadamia nuts, raw	42	Lima	8
		Green split peas	6
		Yellow split peas	5
		Black-eyed peas	4

Soy

Soy is a pretty impressive bean. It contains three times more protein than eggs, and the whole suite of essential amino acids. The global production of soy has increased ten-fold over the past 50 years. Its meal is used in animal feed for hens, cows and pigs. It is also one of the top eight most allergenic foods. This presents a challenge for those who choose to reduce or avoid dairy products, as it is a common replacement. In clinic we find that some children respond positively when soy is removed from their diet. There is even an example of inflammatory markers such as the erythrocyte sedimentation rate (ESR), a measure of how quickly the red blood cells fall to the bottom of a test tube in a sample of blood, which is a measure of inflammation. Some children's ESR level normalizes after removal of soy from the diet.

For those children who do not have a sensitivity to soy, it is preferable to have soy in a more natural form. Edamame beans are a minimally processed example of soy beans. Tofu or tempeh are other examples, rather than more processed versions of soy, such as protein isolates.

Transitioning Proteins

As discussed above, there are many different types of protein that can be chosen. The principles of supernourishing protein sources is that they would be proteins in more of a natural minimally processed state. The types of fats, and the amount of plant nutrient fat protection in the protein, would also need to be considered. The use of chemicals such as herbicides or pesticides, exposure to ocean pollutants, method of cooking, methods of processing and any food sensitivity or allergy can all impact protein selection and overall health value. Adding plant protein to animal protein is a great way to share some of the benefits of plant proteins. Examples of adding plant protein or vegetables to animal protein are given in Chapter 5 with the aim of increasing the overall nutritional value.

Table 3.15: Healthier alternatives for protein sources

Transition out	Replace with
Ham Bacon Sliced meats Frankfurters Canned meats Breaded meats Fried meats Barbecued meat	100% meat Slow-cooked meat Meat cooked at lower heat Grass-fed meats Organic meats Plant proteins or fibre/meat mixes
Tuna	Salmon Sardines Trout
Kidney beans	Cannellini beans Butter beans White beans Lentils Split peas Black-eyed peas (Soaked for 24–48 hours)
Peanuts Salted and roasted nuts	Almonds Macadamia Cashew nuts Seeds
Soy protein	Rice protein Hemp protein

Table 3.15 shows meat, fish, beans, nuts and protein powders that can be divided into two categories. The first column shows proteins that can be transitioned out, and column two shows potential replacements for column one. Transitioning proteins can take time – gradual and consistent efforts are needed.

Fats

Fats are usually divided into three groups according to their structure – monounsaturated, polyunsaturated and saturated. In this section we look at fats in more detail. The structure of the fat only gives us a little bit of information about the overall health value of the fat. We need to know more about whether or not a fat is monounsaturated, polyunsaturated or saturated before we can know whether it is healthy or not.

A rough guide to recognizing healthier fats is that fats that are nearer their natural form tend to be healthier. For example, oils from a whole avocado will be in a healthier, more nutrient-rich medium than extracted oils, even if the oil is virgin avocado oil. Processing an avocado exposes its vulnerable fats to light and oxygen, naturally leading to greater nutrient loss. Even though this is the case, both avocado and its virgin oil are still packed with protective substances such as vitamin E, carotenoids (like beta-carotene) and plant sterols. These protect the fats in the avocado and its oil. If the oil is heated, the natural plant nutrients that it contains are susceptible to damage. So virgin oils are best added after cooking, or heated to a very low heat. Damaged fats have slightly different fat structures when compared to healthy fats, so generally function differently in the body.

Choosing a Variety of Healthy Fats

It is a good idea to eat a variety of fats from foods to give the body all the building blocks it needs for the cell membranes. We saw this in the example of the mitochondrial membrane in Chapter 2. Table 3.16 shows some examples of where you can obtain oils from different groups of fats, and the foods they come from. Preparing fat-rich foods through soaking (where possible), blending and using as dips and dressings in recipes allows these fats to be eaten in a more natural form.

Table 3.16: Healthy sources of oils and fats

Structures	Oils	Foods
Monounsaturated	Extra virgin olive Virgin macadamia Virgin avocado	Guacamole Avocado Olives Nut butters Seed butters Seeds Nuts
Omega-3s	Hemp Flax Fish	Seaweed Smaller fish Hemp seed Flax seeds
Gamma-linolenic acid	Hemp Borage Blackcurrant	Hemp seeds
Medium chain triglycerides	Coconut Coconut butter Sustainably sourced palm	Coconut flour Raw coconut

Cooking with Oils

There are many different lists that recommend the types of fats that you should use in cooking. As a rule, virgin oils should not be used when cooking at very high temperatures that include frying, baking and roasting. This suggests that more highly refined oils should be used for cooking at higher temperatures. There are some suggestions that oils with higher smoking points should be used for cooking at higher temperatures. A smoking point is the temperature that an oil reaches when it begins to continually smoke. When cooking, the oil should not be smoking, as it shows that there is significant breakdown in the structure of the fats. We do not want oils to reach their smoking points when cooking.

Safflower and rice bran oil have the highest smoking points. Ghee has a high smoking point, but is also associated with higher levels of trans fats. Refined or light olive oil and refined coconut oil have higher smoking points. Virgin olive and coconut oil can be used in cooking but at lower temperatures.[90]

PART II
RECIPES

4 Breakfast

Breakfast is the first meal after a night of fasting for 12 hours or more. It provides us with the energy to start the day. During waking and sleep, children use up more energy than adults, and any activity increases energy needs. School is especially demanding due to the sensory stimuli and emotional and learning demands. The stimulating environment – lights, sounds, smells and people – causes glucose use to soar. If your child experiences hypersensitivity to different things like sound, they will experience greater levels of stress, demanding even more glucose. Learning also pushes up glucose requirements, as energy is needed to lay down new neural pathways, to remember how to do a task. A few grams of brain tissue (known as the reticular activating system) is a key player in focusing on tasks, and requires glucose to operate.

Because of this massive glucose demand, it is easy to see why children who skip breakfast may be more vulnerable to distraction and have problems with learning.

Children are particularly prone to low blood sugar, often experiencing symptoms associated with 'hypoglycaemia', before hypoglycemic blood glucose levels are reached. This can directly affect the autonomic nervous system (which regulates internal organs) with symptoms of *tingling, anxiety* or *hunger*. It also can give rise to symptoms such as *dizziness, headaches, inability to concentrate, blurred vision*, and *difficulty speaking* or *walking*. Some of these symptoms may be seen when breakfast is skipped, but can also be seen throughout the day when blood sugar is low. A melt-down or tantrum can sometimes be a sign of lowered blood sugar levels. In clinical practice, some children seem to experience a sudden negative change in behaviour, which is relieved by eating.

Although the results vary, some research suggests that people with autism may use more glucose than people without autism for brain function,[91] whilst other research shows no difference in energy usage. Either way, research shows the positive effects of breakfast on concentration, mood and learning, which makes it important to think about how we time-manage breakfast, and the types of foods we choose.

Grains and Pseudo-Grains

Cereals and breads, pancakes and muffins can have grains as a component. A cereal by definition is a grain used for food, or a breakfast food made from roasted grain and often eaten with milk. Breads, pancakes and muffins are usually made up from a grain flour, although other non-grain flours can be used. Grain normally refers to a species of grass family known as Poaceae. These include the grains listed in Table 4.1 below. We have also listed several pseudo-grains, which are seeds that look similar to grains but are not classed in the same family.

Table 4.1: Gluten-containing and gluten-free grains/pseudo-grains

Gluten-containing grains	Gluten-free grains/pseudo-grains
Wheat, Barley, Rye	Maize
Ancient grains:	Oats
Spelt, Emmer, Farro, Einkorn, Kamut	Millet
Food products made from wheat:	Rice
Durum, Couscous, Semolina, Bulgur wheat	Sorghum
	Teff
	Amaranth
	Wild rice
	Quinoa

Grains are seeds, and as such, are packed full of nutrients for germination and growth. They contain protein storage units known as prolamins. An example of a prolamin is gluten made up of two proteins: gliadin and glutenin. These are naturally quite complex molecules that are difficult to break down. For many centuries we have had different processes for breaking down these proteins before eating them, which include soaking, proofing (for bread), grinding, roasting, boiling and many additional methods. Modern ways of making cereals and breads have sped up this process.

Difficulty in digesting grains also arises from hybridized grains that increase overall protein content. Through industrialization, we now also eat a much larger quantity of grains than ever before.

All these things play a role in why we find it so much more difficult to process grains – not to mention that out gut flora has changed (gut flora plays a significant role in processing proteins).

Using ancient grains or gluten-free grains means that we will typically have fewer plant storage proteins. If we process grains by soaking or sprouting them, this will help. And finally, creating longer processing methods, such as allowing bread to rise for longer, is a good idea.

Breakfasts and Blood Sugar Regulation

Breakfasts vary considerably, from a slice of white toast and jam, to a couple of sausages and tomatoes. As you can imagine, different breakfasts will have different effects on the body. A slice of white toast and jam is more likely to cause glucose levels to spike, resulting in increased levels of circulating insulin. A protein-rich choice, on the other hand, such as sausages and tomatoes, will produce a slow-release response.

The high insulin response to the toast will send the glucose levels plummeting, resulting in blood sugar dips some time during the mid-morning. Mid-morning irritability, loss of concentration and hyperactive behaviour may be observed. Slow-release breakfasts help to slow down the release of glucose into the blood, as well as having an effect on the amount of food needed at lunchtime. This is known as the second meal effect. I have observed that when you help to transition a child from high GI choices to a more protein-rich or lower starch choice of foods, there seems to be a lower need for constant grazing.

Managing blood sugar levels is important because it not only contributes to observable behaviour changes, but it also influences the brain processing we spoke about in Chapter 1. The brain is in a constant state of flux and is influenced by factors such as infections, food sensitivity and also blood sugar fluctuations. Any of these factors can drive inflammation, influencing processing ability and resulting in slower comprehension of instructions or ability to carry out a task. For all these reasons, careful thought and planning is important on our journey towards healthier breakfasts.

For the sake of simplicity, let's split breakfasts into three groups: first, cereals; second, bread, pancakes and muffins; and third, non-grain-based breakfasts.

Cereals

Cereals vary in nutritional content. For example, 30g of sugared cornflakes without milk contains 13.2g of sugar. The equivalent amount of rolled oats (30g) contains 0g of sugar. Oats have 13 times more fibre than the sugared cornflakes, and 11 times more magnesium (essential for processing carbohydrates to make energy). The sugared cornflakes are fortified, so contain higher levels of calcium and B vitamins, although those B vitamins that occur naturally in food have a broader spectrum of forms than those added during fortification.

Whatever you add to cereal will affect its overall nutritional value (your blood sugar can also be affected by choices made – see page 29). If, for example, you replace 3 teaspoons of cornflakes with 3 teaspoons of ground almonds in a bowl of 35g of cornflakes, you can increase its overall protein by 30 per cent, reduce its carbohydrate content by 25 per cent, and increase its fat by 85 per cent. This will reduce the overall GI by 20 per cent, and triple the fibre levels.

It may seem like a little change, but these changes, multiplied over a week, help to contribute to improve nutrient density and glycaemic control. Little changes like this can help to transition a child into healthier foods.

You could add the following to cereals to increase fibre and nutrient density: 1 teaspoon of flaxseed, coconut flour, almond flour, sunflower seeds, pumpkin seeds or coconut flakes or desiccated coconut. If need be, start with even smaller quantities.

In the next section we present a range of recipes for breakfast. It is hoped that some will encourage you to make such changes.

RAW FOOD PORRIDGE

Gluten-free • Grain-free • Dairy-free • Casein-free • Low oxalate (option) • Low FODMAP

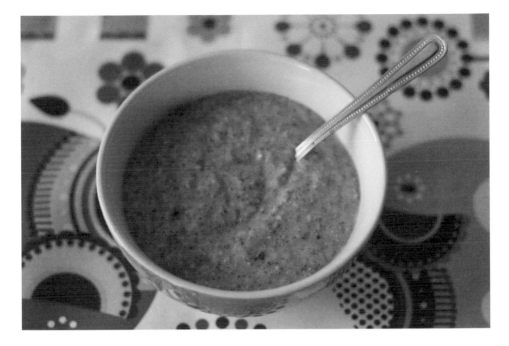

This porridge is super simple to make, and is grain-free. It is also naturally sweetened by the apple, so you only need to add in the dates for extra sweetness.

300ml (2 cups) coconut milk or milk of your choice

1 green apple, grated

2 tbsp chia seeds (extremely high in oxalate and phenol)

2 tbsp desiccated coconut

2 dates, roughly chopped (optional)

½ tsp ground cinnamon

1 Warm the milk in a saucepan.

2 Transfer the warm milk to a mixing bowl.

3 Add the grated apple.

4 Add the remaining ingredients.

5 Blend until mixed together.

This can be prepared the night before, and then warmed up in the morning.

BUTTERNUT SQUASH AND PAPAYA MILLET PORRIDGE

Gluten-free • Dairy-free • Casein-free • Low phenol (moderate) • Low oxalate (option) • Low FODMAP

This porridge is packed full of carotenoids that help to protect cell membranes and blood vessels. It is easy on the stomach, and as the millet is blended, it is easier to digest, especially if it is soaked overnight.

½ butternut squash

½ papaya

170ml (1 cup) coconut milk or milk of your choice

140g (1 cup) cooked millet

1 tsp cinnamon (high oxalate) (optional)

1 tsp vanilla extract

1 Preheat the oven to 175°C/350°F/gas mark 4.

2 Chop the butternut squash in half, remove the seeds, and bake for 35–50 minutes or until tender (depending on its size).

3 Once the butternut squash has cooled down, scoop the flesh out.

4 Blend the butternut squash with the remaining ingredients.

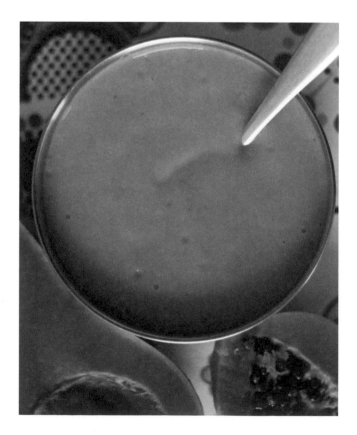

Breads, Pancakes and Muffins

Bread is called the 'staff of life'. Wheat flour, because of its high gluten content, creates amazing texture, giving bread its characteristic chewiness. The bread, pancake and muffin recipes that follow are easy to make, grain-free, soaked, lower GI and supernourishing.

Muffins and pancakes are easy options. It is also easy to sneak in vegetables or fruits. Begin with a small amount of vegetables, and then work your way up. Try adding vegetables to foods on one day, and then make a plain pancake or muffin on another day. You want to be unpredictable, otherwise if there is a pattern of adding vegetables it increases the chances that your child will reject the muffin or pancake with the vegetable.

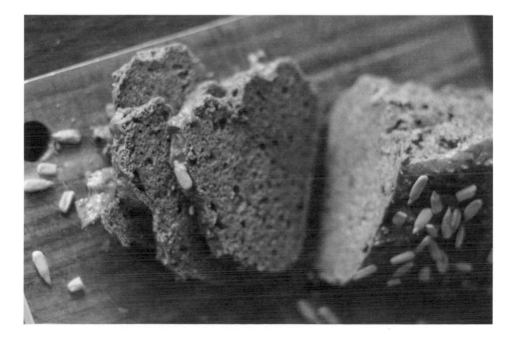

SUNFLOWER BUTTER BREAD

Gluten-free • Grain-free • Dairy-free • Casein-free • SCD • GAPS • Low phenol • Low oxalate (thinly sliced) • Low FODMAP

Sunflower Butter Bread is an easy, very low carbohydrate option that is grain-, nut-, yeast- and dairy-free. Sunflower butter is also a lower oxalate choice. Two tablespoons of sunflower butter is considered to contain moderate levels of oxalate. This bread contains about 8 tablespoons. So if the bread is divided into ten slices or more, one slice would have a low to moderate amount of oxalate. The bread is flexible and should not be too crumbly if it is mixed well. It makes a good sandwich bread.

Sunflower seeds are a rich source of vitamin E and phytosterols, and are protective to fats in the body.

250g (1 cup) sunflower butter (room temperature)

3 eggs (separate the yolks from the whites)

1 tbsp apple cider vinegar

¼ tsp sea salt

½ tsp baking powder

½ tsp bicarbonate of soda

1 Pre-heat the oven to 175°C/350°F/gas mark 4.

2 Combine the sunflower butter with the egg yolks, cider vinegar, sea salt, baking powder and bicarbonate of soda, using a wooden spoon. This should take a few minutes.

3 Beat the egg whites for about 1 minute, then add to the other mixture, and combine them together until thoroughly mixed in.

4 Line the bottom of a bread/loaf tin with parchment paper.

5 Spoon the mixture into the bread tin.

6 Bake for 35–40 minutes or until cooked through. The timing may vary slightly depending on the oven temperature and type of oven. Check using a knife or skewer – when inserted into the loaf, it should come out clean.

7 Remove the bread from the oven and leave it to cool on a cooling rack.

8 The loaf can be sliced and frozen, or put in a plastic bag and kept in the fridge for 3–4 days.

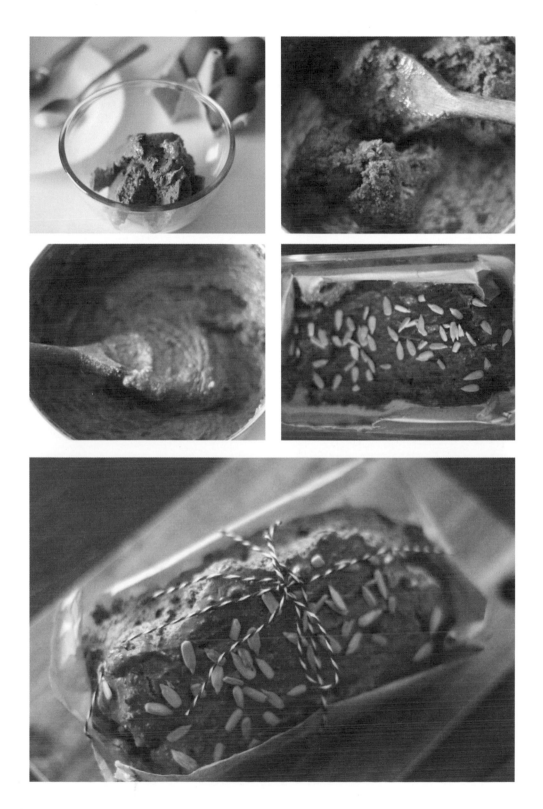

GERMINATED BROWN (WHOLEGRAIN) RICE

We will be using germinated brown rice in the Egg-Free Fermented Rice Pancakes recipe.

Many cultures around the world soak rice and other grains, and for good reason. Science has finally caught up, showing that soaking helps to reduce phytates (also known as anti-nutrients) that can bind to minerals, and activates nutrients and helps to make the grain easier to digest.

Soaking the rice creates a tiny sprout. Following germination, the nutrient concentration in the wholegrain rice is at its maximum. The nutrients include vitamins B1, B3, B6, E, magnesium, potassium and zinc, and the amino acid lysine (which has an anti-viral effect). Gamma-aminobutyric acid (GABA), a calming brain chemical, is increased in rice after soaking at about 40°C for 8–24 hours. GABA has been associated with improved sleep and activation of intestinal motility in the gut, so may also be helpful with constipation. It is also helpful for anxiety.[92]

120–140g (1–2 cups) cooked brown rice

1 Soak the rice overnight, at room temperature.

2 Place the soaked rice in the fridge and leave for another 24 hours.

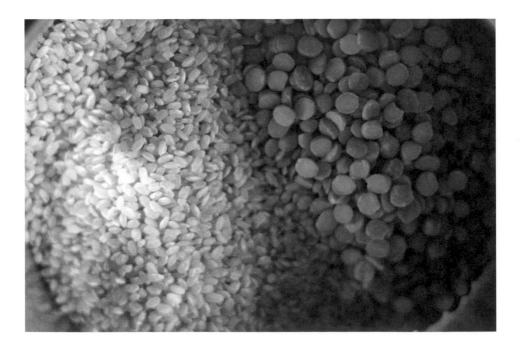

EGG-FREE FERMENTED RICE PANCAKES (LOW GI)

Gluten-free • Dairy-free • Casein-free • Low phenol • Low oxalate • Low FODMAP

This is one of the simplest egg-free pancakes you will come across. It is made from brown short-grain rice and split peas (chana dhal), rather than brown rice flour, so the GI is lower.

The good thing about these pancakes is that they are gluten-, nut- and egg-free. They also are low in oxalate. Some children do not tolerate processed rice products well, but do tolerate rice in its natural form (such as cooked brown rice).

150g (1 cup) yellow dried split peas (chana dal)

180g (2 cups) brown short-grain rice

60–125ml (¼–½ cup) water

Pinch of salt

1 tbsp organic rice bran oil

1 Soak the split peas and rice without any salt (as it slows the fermentation process) for up to 48 hours. Change the water every four hours. You can put them in the fridge after one day of soaking.

2 Rinse and drain.

3 Blend the split peas, rice, water and salt together, until the mixture is smooth.

4 Leave to stand for about 15 minutes, and then add enough water until the mixture has a dropping consistency.

5 Add the rice bran oil to the saucepan and allow to warm, then pour 2–3 tbsp of the batter into the pan until it lightly coats the base. Cook for about 1½ minutes, until it sets.

6 Slip a palette knife under the crepe and flip it. Cook on the other side for about 30 seconds.

Non-Grain Breakfasts

Non-grain breakfasts don't usually contain breads or cereals. Examples include yoghurt and fruit, or the British breakfast (without potatoes or toast). These choices tend to be much lower in carbohydrates and higher in protein.

FLOURLESS PANCAKES

Gluten-free • Grain-free• Dairy-free • Casein-free • SCD • GAPS •
Low phenol • Low oxalate (moderate) • Low FODMAP

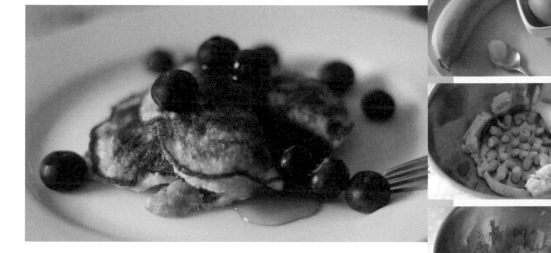

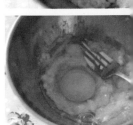

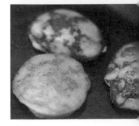

These are packed with protein and have a low GI.

1 egg
1 banana, mashed
¼ tsp bicarbonate of soda
½ tsp cinnamon
½ tsp ginger

1 Whisk the egg in a bowl.

2 Add the mashed banana.

3 Add the bicarbonate of soda and mix well.

4 Add cinnamon and ginger if using.

British Breakfast

A high-protein diet can be a helpful option for some children. This is because protein is the best nutrient out of protein, fat and carbohydrates for slowing down sugar release, which leads to more balanced blood sugar levels throughout the day. I have found that some children do not graze as much with a high-protein breakfast.

The British breakfast is classically a very high-protein option. It typically consists of bacon, sausages and eggs, often with added baked beans, mushrooms and hash browns. The meat and eggs are often fried in fat. If no beans are added, the breakfast is also low in fibre.

To improve the overall nutrient density of the British breakfast, consider the following options:

- Use homemade sausages/patties.

- Omit the bacon.

- Have poached eggs instead of fried eggs.

- Have grilled mushrooms, tomatoes and avocados.

- Omit the hash browns, or make them out of sweet potato or courgette (zucchini) (see recipes below).

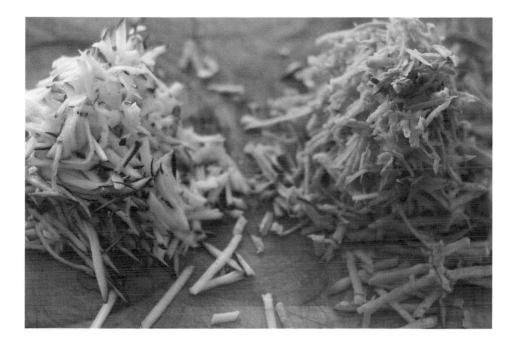

SWEET POTATO HASH BROWNS

Gluten-free • Grain-free • Dairy-free • Casein-free • Low FODMAP

1 medium-sized sweet potato

Pinch of salt

1 tbsp olive oil

1 Grate the sweet potato.

2 Stir-fry the sweet potato with a pinch of salt in the oil for 5 minutes.

COURGETTE (ZUCCHINI) HASH BROWNS

Gluten-free • Grain-free • Dairy-free • Casein-free • SCD • GAPS • Low phenol • Low oxalate • Low FODMAP

1 medium courgette (zucchini)

½ onion, finely chopped

Pinch of salt

1 tbsp olive oil

1 Grate the courgette (peel it for a lower phenol option).

2 Stir-fry the courgette and chopped onion in the oil, with the salt, for 3–5 minutes.

BREAKFAST SAUSAGE

Gluten-free • Grain-free • Dairy-free • Casein-free • SCD • GAPS • Low phenol (option) • Low oxalate • Low FODMAP

225g (2 cups) organic turkey

2 tbsp lettuce pulp (from juicing)

2 tbsp sage (or omit this for low phenol)

1 tbsp fresh rosemary (or omit this for low phenol)

1½ tsp sea salt

1 tbsp olive oil

1 Grind the turkey in a food processor or use turkey mince (ground meat) instead.

2 Add the lettuce pulp, sage and rosemary (if using), and salt.

3 Using an ice-cream scoop, take out one scoop and shape into a round. Continue until you've made 4–6 patties.

4 Heat the olive oil in a large frying pan or skillet, and fry each pattie for 8–10 minutes, then turn over and fry for a further 8 minutes on the other side.

CASHEW NUT MILK YOGHURT

Gluten-free • Grain-free • Dairy-free • Casein-free • SCD • GAPS • Low FODMAP

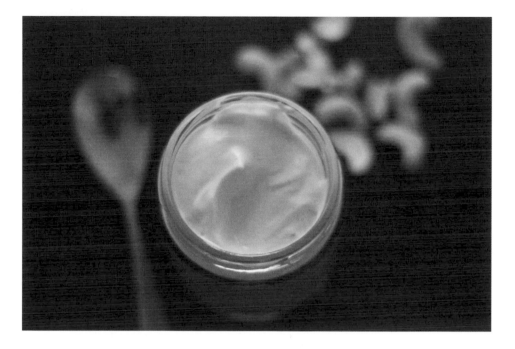

125g (1 cup) cashew nuts

125ml (½ cup) water (plus extra for desired consistency)

1 SCD- and GAPS-compliant probiotic capsule

1 Soak the cashew nuts overnight.

2 Rinse and drain.

3 Blend the cashew nuts with the water and probiotic.

4 Leave the mixture overnight and then refrigerate.

BLUEBERRY AND AVOCADO YOGHURT

Gluten-free • Grain-free • Dairy-free • Casein-free • SCD • GAPS • High polyol FODMAP

200g (2 cups)
blueberries

½ avocado

1 SCD- and GAPS-
compliant probiotic
capsule

1 Blend all the ingredients together.

2 Refrigerate overnight.

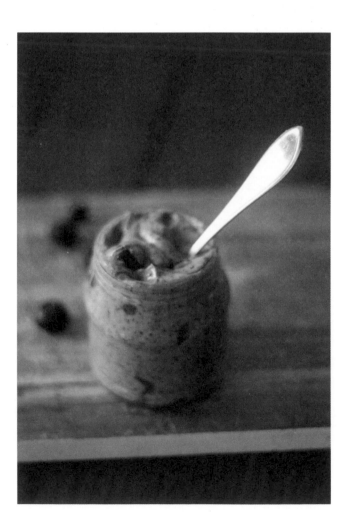

ALMOND MILK

Gluten-free • Grain-free • Dairy-free • Casein-free • SCD • GAPS • Low FODMAP

35g (1 cup) almonds
750ml (3 cups) water
1 tsp sunflower lecithin

1 Soak the almonds overnight.

2 Rinse and drain.

3 Blend the almonds with half of the water, until smooth.

4 Add the remaining water and continue to blend.

5 Pass the mixture through a muslin cloth.

6 Refrigerate.

7 You can add sunflower lecithin to prevent the almond milk from separating when left to stand.

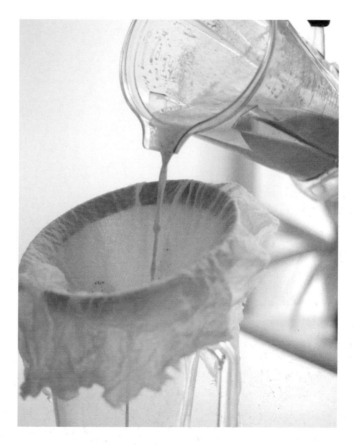

5 Lunch

Lunch is considered to be the most important meal of the day in some European countries. In other places, it is a rushed affair – eating on the run, in the car, on the street, or rushing in the school's cafeteria or hall.

Rushing does not help the digestive process. This is because rushing usually promotes stress and shuts down the nerve and hormonal rhythms that aid digestion. Rushing also means that food is not chewed well, so the food will not be broken down, making it more difficult to digest.

At schools the lunchtime period can be especially stressful. Stimulation can stress a child with heightened sensory issues, for example, the smell of food cooking, flickering from fluorescent lights, constant conversation and rising noise 'reverberating from...cafeteria walls'.[93]

Social inclusion is also important. As a parent, the challenge is that the food your child has in their packed lunch may look quite different to everyone else's. Your child may also grab food that looks more desirable from other children's plates or lunch boxes.

Homemade school lunches need more planning time and preparation, and don't have the convenience of a quick sandwich or shop-bought snacks. Let's begin by looking at typical lunchtime meal choices.

From a nutritional perspective, the ideal lunch would be rich in phytonutrients from fruits or vegetables, whole plant foods including wholegrains, quality protein, and minimally processed fats. This type of lunch helps to keep up the after-lunch energy levels, and helps your child navigate the natural daily dip that occurs in the early afternoon and might make them feel sleepy. Here are several tips to help increase the nutritional density of lunchtime options.

Transitioning Towards Healthier Lunches

1. With 'picky' eaters, start small, making little changes (see Table 5.1).

Table 5.1: Transition ideas for healthier lunch options

Current lunch options	Transition ideas
White bread sandwich with ham	Add 1 tsp psyllium husk to the spread, to increase fibre
Ham, cheese or processed meat slices	Use leftovers from a roasted chicken, or buy 100% meat, sliced
Potato crisps	Vegetable crisps
Box of raisins or dried fruit	Fresh fruit
No vegetables	Carrot sticks Lightly steamed French beans
Shop-bought biscuits	Homemade biscuits

2. Gluten-free products can be lower in fibre. Adding high-fibre foods to sandwiches can increase overall fibre content. You could choose a brown version of gluten-free bread – sometimes this will mean the bread has almost twice as much fibre in each slice. Other options include adding:

   - 1 tsp whole chia – 1.3g fibre

   - ½ tsp psyllium husk – 2.5g fibre

   - 1 iceberg lettuce portion (25g or ½ cup) – 0.3g fibre

   - 1 tsp hummus – 0.4g fibre

   - 2 tsp sunflower seeds – 0.4g fibre

   - 1 tsp pumpkin seed butter – 0.3g fibre

3. You may have heard of the open sandwich. This is when you only eat one side of a bread sandwich. Try this by only making half a round of sandwiches, replacing the other half with nutrient-dense options (see Table 5.2).

Table 5.2: Nutrient-dense lunchtime options

Food	Nutrient-dense options
Meat	Use 100% meat Chop into chunks or roll up slices
Legumes	Edamame (soya beans) French beans (lightly steamed) Sugar snap beans (lightly steamed) Mange tout (snow peas) (lightly steamed)
Vegetables	Carrot sticks Organic celery Red pepper slices
Fruit	Fresh grapes Fresh blueberries Fresh organic strawberries Sliced apple (mixed with lemon juice to reduce any discolouration) Sliced plums Chopped mango Chopped papaya

Introducing homemade foods is often a challenge when children with autism are used to eating their favourite shop-bought brands. I suggest that if your child has an ABA therapist who understands how to introduce new foods, then you begin the introduction at home. Sometimes a child will sample new foods at school, but not at home.

Muffins	Homemade (see recipes)
Biscuits	Homemade (see recipes)
Bread or pancake as a wrap	Homemade (see recipes)
Crackers	Homemade (see recipes)
Smoothies	Make one of the homemade supernutritious smoothies, with a little protein powder as an option

4. If you are replacing options in your child's packed lunch box, or if your child needs an extra few calories, why not try adding in extra portions from the list in Table 5.3?

Table 5.3: Food choices with calories

Food choice	Energy (Kcal)
½ chicken breast, chopped up (grilled, skin removed)	74
2 tbsp green beans (add an oil-based dressing to this)	13.2
4 slices cucumber (dip in mayonnaise, or make an oil-based dressing)	4.5
½ medium carrot, chopped into sticks	11.7
Add an oil-based dressing:	
2 tsp mayonnaise	90
1 tbsp hummus	89
1 tbsp guacamole	45
1 tsp coconut oil	33
1 tsp virgin avocado oil	36

You can add the condiments or dips to the bread before you add the sandwich filling – for example, adding mayonnaise increases the calorific and nutrient value. If you are replacing a slice of bread, remember that an average slice of bread contains about 75–85 Kcal.

5. Make a note of what is coming home in the lunch box to see if your child is choosing the nutrient-dense choices in their lunch box. If not, continue with the standard lunch, and work with the ABA therapist or feeding therapist to increase nutrient-dense options.

Neophobia (Fear of Trying New Things, Including Foods)

When a new food is introduced to a child, it may take ten tries for them to get used to it. In children with autism, with their heightened sense of flavours, textures and possible negative experiences with food, it may take up to and sometimes more than 30 tries.

6. Choose quality proteins. Processed meats can be defined as 'any meat preserved by smoking, curing, salting or adding preservatives'. Examples of these types of meat include bacon, ham, salami, hot dogs and pastrami. These types of meats tend to have higher levels of salt and fat.[94] Transition protein choices towards:

- 100% meat slices
- Grilled whole meats (low heat)
- Smaller fish (e.g. salmon)
- Beans and bean dips (e.g. hummus)
- French beans with dips like mayonnaise
- Coconut-based vegan cheeses
- Eggs (boiled)
- Soft cheeses (ricotta, goat's cheese, if tolerated)

LUNCHTIME RICE BOWL

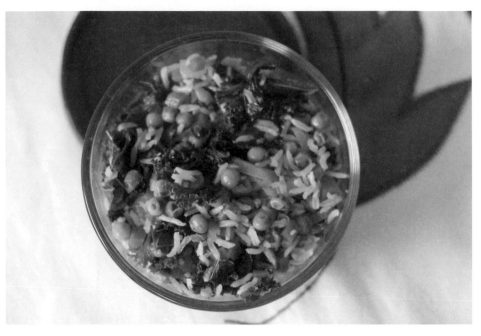

The idea behind a lunchtime rice bowl is that it can be quick and easy to make. It can be eaten cold or kept in a thermal flask. The base of it can have rice, quinoa, millet, buckwheat, or whatever grain you choose. The key factor is that you choose a wholegrain, or at least add in some wholegrain if transitioning from white rice, or add some Veggie Rice (see recipes below).

You can make these rice bowls one to two days in advance. This could be done on a Sunday and Wednesday evening, changing choices with each batch you put together.

See Table 5.4 for different ingredient options

1 Choose a grain base from the list in Table 5.4.

2 Soak overnight (or for 48 hours).

3 Cook the grains using the amount of water in the table. Some of the grains need cooking for a specific time, and then you can add 5 minutes with the pan lid on to allow the grain to steam for 5 more minutes.

4 Choose a handful of vegetables from the list.

5 Choose a handful of protein from the list.

6 Add three teaspoons of dressing – add high-quality fats or a dressing from the list.

Table 5.4: Rice bowl options

Grain	Water (cups)	Amount (cups)	Time (mins)	Yield (cups)
Buckwheat, unroasted	2	1	15–20	3½
Millet	1²/₃	1	30 + 5 steam	3
Quinoa	1²/₃	1	15 + 5 steam	3
Teff	2½–3	1	20	1
Wholegrain rice	1¾	1	45	2

Vegetables

Steamed, cooked or grilled	Raw
Courgette (zucchini)	Red peppers
Broccoli	Carrots
Carrots	Spring onions (scallions)
Kale	Rocket
Cabbage	Watercress
Pumpkin	Lamb's lettuce
Butternut squash	
Shredded cabbage	

Protein

Chicken, salmon, green beans, peas, lentils, split peas, chickpeas

Dressing

Coconut oil, virgin avocado oil, virgin macadamia oil, hemp oil

Veggie Rice

The idea behind veggie rice is simple. Chop or grate vegetables into small rice-sized bits. Sneak these into the rice, or eat as an alternative to rice, with some higher calorie choices. You can also try making a 50/50 rice bowl, adding stir-fried vegetables for a quick lunchtime meal.

Cauliflower is an easy-to-disguise option due to its colour and how it grates into little pieces. It has a strong flavour, however, so you might need to mask it with tomato or another strong seasoning.

CAULIFLOWER RICE

Gluten-free • Grain-free • Dairy-free • Casein-free • SCD • GAPS • Low oxalate • High polyol FODMAP

Cauliflower rice is a good alternative for lots of reasons. First, it keeps you regular. Cauliflower contains a little-known sugar called a polyol (see Chapter 3). Polyols help movement in the gut. The combination of short-grain rice with cauliflower is a recipe for 'bowel movement'. The polyols in cauliflower are mini alcohol sugars that act as a laxative, and the short-grain rice acts as a bulking agent.

1 cauliflower

1 tbsp oil of your choice

1 Grate the whole cauliflower head (but do not grate the stalks as these can be bitter).

2 Stir-fry the cauliflower for 3–4 minutes in the oil.

CAULIFLOWER RICE COMBO

180g (1 cup) short-grain rice

1 portion Cauliflower Rice (see recipe)

1 Cook the short-grain rice separately, for 35–45 minutes, or until tender and fluffy.

2 Add in the Cauliflower Rice.

Cauliflower has about six times more fibre, gram for gram, compared to rice. It contains one of the lowest GI levels of the typical vegetables used in grain-free diets. You may need to begin by adding a small amount of cauliflower to the rice, building up the amount up slowly.

EGG-FRIED CAULIFLOWER RICE

Gluten-free • Grain-free • Dairy-free • Casein-free • SCD • GAPS • Low oxalate •
High polyol FODMAP

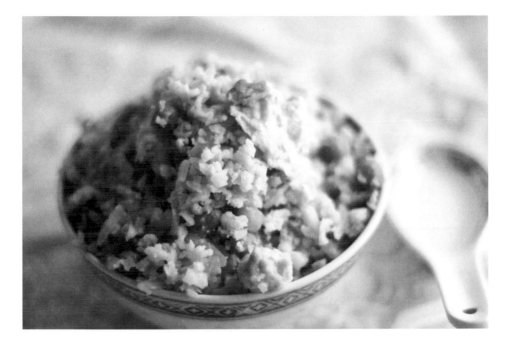

Egg-fried rice is usually made with long-grain rice, but this recipe uses short-grain rice. It is super-quick to make, as you do not need to cook the cauliflower in advance.

1 cauliflower
1 spring onion (scallion)
140g (1 cup) peas
1 tbsp oil of your choice
1–2 eggs
Pinch of salt

1 Grate the whole cauliflower (omitting the stalk).

2 Chop the spring onion. If there are salicylate issues, just use the white part of the spring onion, or try golden onions instead.

3 Put the spring onion in a pan with the peas and oil, and stir-fry for 1–2 minutes.

4 Add the grated cauliflower and stir-fry for 3–4 minutes, or until the cauliflower is tender.

5 Beat the eggs, and then scramble them in a separate pan.

6 Add the eggs to the cauliflower rice and stir through.

Breadless 'sandwiches'

Sandwiches are one of the easiest and quickest lunches to make. The bigger challenge is how to make a sandwich-like meal without bread. Below are some ideas to get you started.

A 'breadless sandwich' is a nutrient-dense food in a lunch box. I got the idea from Prêt à Manger (a sandwich shop) in the UK. They have little sandwich-size lunch boxes with sandwich-like fillings, vegetables and no bread. Table 5.5 below shows four different options for a no-bread sandwich. Portion sizes should be adjusted for the age of the child.

Table 5.5: Different options for a breadless sandwich

Protein (choose 1–2)	Green leafy vegetable (choose 1)	Dressing/dip (choose 1)	Extra vegetables (choose 2–3)
Chicken/turkey	Cos lettuce	Mayonnaise	Cooked butternut squash
Sliced lamb (lean)	Iceberg lettuce (organic)	Guacamole	Cooked pumpkin
Egg or ricotta	Rocket	Ranch dressing (dairy-free)	Cooked sweet potato
Salmon	Butter	Yoghurt	Cucumber
Hummus/dip	Lamb's lettuce	Tzatziki (dairy-free)	Carrot sticks
Almond hummus/ nut dip	Batavia lettuce	Nut 'no peanut' dressing	Tomato

You can add different dips or dressings to the lunchtime option, as mentioned earlier. Here are some recipes for you to try.

LETTUCE FAJITA

Gluten-free • Grain-free • Dairy-free • Casein-free • SCD • GAPS • Low oxalate •
High polyol FODMAP

Parchment paper can be used to hold these fajitas in place.

½ onion

1 tbsp virgin olive oil

½ pepper (omit if there is a phenol/salicylate sensitivity)

1 chicken breast, cut into strips

Cos, romaine or butter lettuce

¼ avocado, mashed (omit if there is a phenol/salicylate sensitivity)

1 tsp mayonnaise

1 Slice the onion and pepper, and sauté in the oil on a very low heat for a few minutes.

2 Grill the chicken breast strips.

3 Take two lettuce leaves, and lay them on a plate.

4 Put the mashed avocado and mayonnaise on top of each lettuce leaf.

5 Add three strips of chicken, with a few pieces of onion and pepper.

6 Pinch two sides of the lettuce leaves together with the filling inside, and wrap with parchment paper to hold.

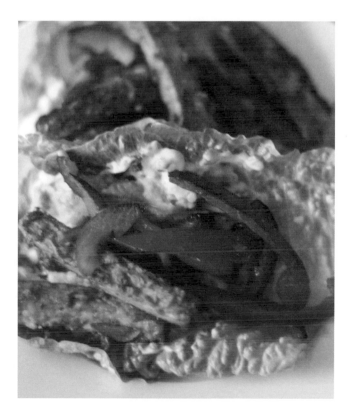

Dips and Dressings
DAIRY-FREE RANCH DRESSING

Gluten-free • Grain-free • Dairy-free • Casein-free • SCD • GAPS • Low phenol •
Low FODMAP

125g (1 cup) cashew nuts, soaked overnight

185ml (¾ cup) water

Juice of ½ lemon

60ml (¼ cup) organic apple cider vinegar

60ml (¼ cup) extra virgin olive oil

A few leaves of basil, chives and dill, finely chopped

1 tsp sea salt

1 Blend all the ingredients together, apart from the herbs.

2 Once the mixture is blended, add the herbs.

MACADAMIA HUMMUS

Gluten-free • Grain-free • Dairy-free • Casein-free • SCD • GAPS • Low FODMAP

This recipe is inspired by the recipe from *Plant Food*.[95]

180g (1 cup) courgette (zucchini), peeled

60g (½ cup) macadamia nuts, soaked for 2 hours

120ml (½ cup) tahini

120ml (½ cup) extra virgin olive oil

60ml (¼ cup) lemon juice

1 tsp cumin seeds

1 clove of garlic, crushed

1 tsp sea salt

1 Blend all the ingredients together.

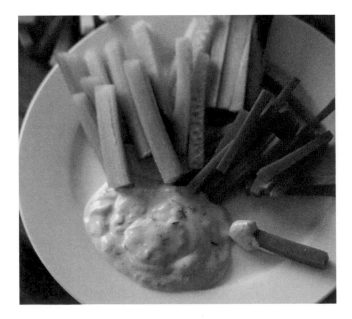

Noodles

Home-cooked lunches need to be quick. Noodles are quick and easy. There are many different types of noodles available that are gluten-free. Even if you do not normally choose gluten-free options, it is a good idea to increase variety in the diet to rotate the types of grains (noodles) that you eat. This allows for a more varied diet. Noodles vary in nutritional density – some are very starchy and low in nutrients whilst others, like buckwheat noodles, tend to be more nutrient-packed.

Table 5.6: Different noodle options

Noodles	Description
Buckwheat (soba)	Chewy noodles, quite strong tasting
Kelp	Made from seaweed, relatively flavourless
Rice (can have mixes of rice and another ingredient such as millet)	Soft-textured noodles
Arrowroot	Like a vermicelli noodle – can look a little glassy when cooked
Mung bean starch	Glass noodles are see-through; they have to be cooked for quite a while
Rice	Soft-textured noodles
Shirataki	Noodles made from a tuber vegetable called konjac, which is low in carbohydrate
Sweet potato	This is sweet potato starch

Vegetable noodles

Vegetable noodles are vegetables turned into noodles using a spiralizer (see below). Courgette (zucchini), sweet potatoes, parsnips, carrots and butternut squash can all be turned into noodles. For children who do not like colours or flavours, courgettes are a good option, especially if they are peeled. Vegetable noodles can be stir-fried or steamed, and they can be added to any grain-based cooked noodle or pasta. If you do not have a spiralizer, you can use a vegetable peeler to create strips of vegetables that can also be steamed or stir-fried.

Using a spiralizer

A spiralizer is pretty easy to use, with a little practice.

1. Wash the vegetable. Courgettes (zucchini) are ideal as they do not need to be chopped to size to fit the spiralizer.

2. Attach one end of the courgette to the end of the spiralizer with the blade. There is a small metal cylinder that you can attach the courgette to.

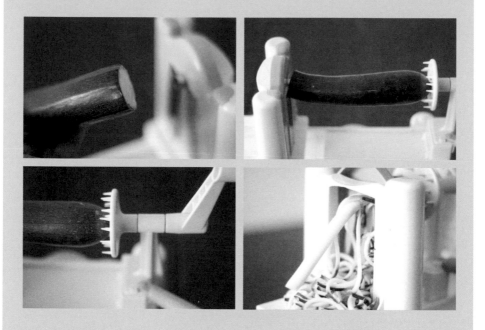

3. Press the round thing with the bits sticking out into the end of the courgette.

4. Turn the handle.

5. Slide the spiralizer slowly, using one of your hands.

6. Spiralize the vegetable.

COURGETTE (ZUCCHINI) 'SPAGHETTI' NEAPOLITAN

Gluten-free • Grain-free • Dairy-free • Casein-free • SCD • GAPS • Low phenol • Low oxalate • Low FODMAP

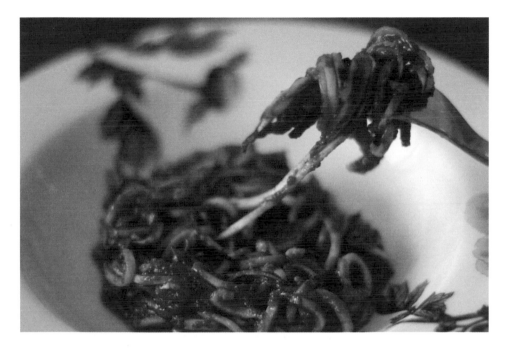

1 courgette (zucchini)

3 tbsp tomato purée (omit tomatoes for a low phenol option)

6 tbsp water

1 tbsp extra virgin olive oil

Pinch of dried oregano

Pinch of salt

Pinch of garlic powder or 1 clove garlic, crushed

1 Spiralize the courgette.

2 You can cook the spiralized courgette in one of two ways: either use what I call the *stir-dry* method – heat a wok under a medium flame, add the courgette to the wok and stir, without adding any water or oil. Alternatively, *stir-steam* – add 1–2 tbsp of water, cover the courgettes for 1–2 minutes and let them steam.

3 Combine all the remaining ingredients, then add to the courgette and stir in the wok for another 1–2 minutes.

Other Lunch Ideas
BROCCOLI AND PEA CREAM SOUP

Gluten-free • Grain-free • Dairy-free • Casein-free • SCD • GAPS • Low oxalate •
Low FODMAP

The amazing thing about broccoli and pea cream soup is that it's creamy without the cream. When you blend broccoli, it creates a creamy consistency. Adding in a blended pulse or bean increases the creaminess even further. Peas, split peas and cannellini beans are all options that blend well with broccoli. Both beans and vegetables are low in calories, so adding extra calories is a good idea. This can be done by adding 1 teaspoon of virgin oil to the soup, and serving it with bread, or other options such as cooked wholegrain rice, simply adding sweet potatoes for texture, or a nut cream, such as Cashew Nut Cream.

This Broccoli and Pea Cream Soup is one of the simplest soups to make; from the chopping board to the table it takes about 10 minutes (if you're quick, and with practice!).

1.5 litres (6 cups) water

Stock cube (optional) or ½ tsp sea salt

1 broccoli head (you could exchange the broccoli for Brussels sprouts or white cabbage for a low phenol option)

280g (2 cups) peas

1 Bring the water to the boil, and add a stock cube or salt.

2 Separate the broccoli florets into small pieces, and add to the boiling water along with the peas.

3 Boil for 3–5 minutes, or until the broccoli is cooked.

4 Blend everything together to make the soup.

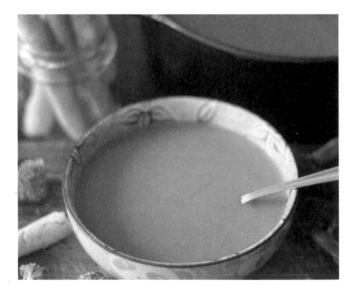

CASHEW NUT CREAM

Gluten-free • Grain-free • Dairy-free • Casein-free • SCD • GAPS • Low phenol •
Low FODMAP

Cashew nuts are a great culinary substitute for normal cream because they are
very starchy for a nut. This makes them good for thickening soups or for making
creamy sauces.

100g (1 cup) cashew
nuts, soaked for a
minimum of 2 hours to
overnight

60ml (¼ cup) water

Juice of ½ large lemon

Pinch of sea salt

1 Blend the soaked cashew nuts, water, lemon juice and
sea salt, until you get the desired consistency.

SWEDE (RUTABAGAS) CHIPS

Gluten-free • Grain-free • Dairy-free • Casein-free • SCD • GAPS • Low phenol •
Low oxalate • Low FODMAP

Swede is a low-carbohydrate vegetable that can be used to make oven fries or
chips. You can add swede chips to the fries that your child normally eats, although
they do generally like to pick them out. Swedes have an earthy taste, with a tiny
hint of bitterness at the end. Potatoes are much milder in flavour – 100g of potato
yields 17g of carbohydrate, whereas 100g of swede contains 2.3g. The flavour of
swede is slightly sweeter than potatoes, with slightly more sugars – 2.2g in swede
versus 1.4g in potatoes. Swede also has a higher water content, and with the
much lower carbohydrate content, will not get crisp like potatoes. Getting your
children to rub the oil into the swede can be a good way to help introduce them
to the vegetable.

1 medium swede

½–1 tbsp olive oil

1 Peel the swede.

2 Slice into chip-shaped sizes.

3 Mix the swede with the olive oil.

4 Bake in the oven at 200ºC/400ºF/gas mark 6 for
40–50 minutes, and serve immediately.

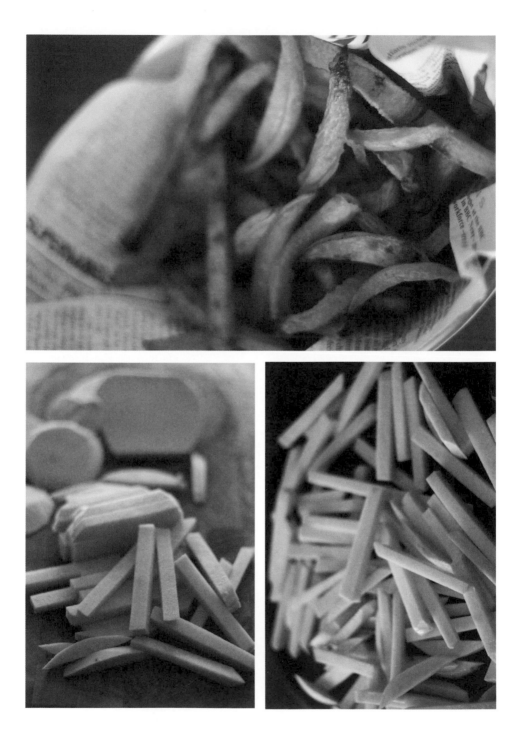

PIZZA BASE

Gluten-free • Dairy-free • Casein-free • Low FODMAP

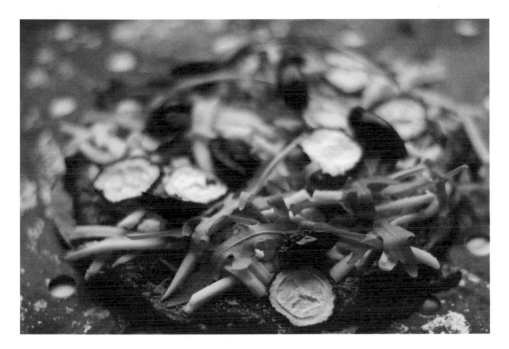

135g (¾ cup) wholegrain rice

30g (¼ cup) chia seeds

¼ tsp bicarbonate of soda

60ml (¼ cup) water, for blending

1 Soak the rice and chia seeds overnight in separate bowls, and then rinse and drain.

2 Blend all the ingredients together.

3 Take 3 tbsp of the mixture and spread it on a lined baking tray, in a circular shape.

4 Bake for 15 minutes or until firm.

5 Add toppings of your choice (e.g. tomato sauce, olives, sweetcorn, peppers, garlic, protein choices).

6 Dinner

Dinner is usually the last meal before bedtime, and it is probably the meal that needs the most planning to coordinate the different dietary preferences of the family.

In this chapter there are ideas to increase the variety of dinnertime options. We look at increasing vegetable intake as a main theme, whilst trying to maximize nutrients, increase fibre and reduce overall GI.

Battle of the mash

Mashed potato is a comfort food, creamy smooth and fluffy, made with floury King Edward or Maris Piper potatoes for the best results. (Don't make the mistake of using a hand blender as you will end up with gluey mashed potato.)

When it comes to vegetable mash, the rules change. Many vegetables have a much higher water to starch ratio than white potatoes, so the mash can turn out watery. A combination of high water content, low carbohydrate and low fibre are not the best formula for an alternative to mashed potato. I think the most important ingredient in a good mash is the carbohydrate content/fibre content, so let's look at the battle for a potato mash alternative, and see what wins.

Table 6.1: Mashed vegetable alternatives

Vegetable	Amount	Time to cook (mins)	Textures and flavours
Carrot	2 medium carrots	15–20	Sweet, hard, a little watery
Cauliflower	¼ cauliflower	5–10	Soft, a bit watery
Celeriac	1 large celeriac	25–30	Lots of fibre, strong celery taste, even after adding something like butter
Parsnip	2 medium-sized parsnips	20	Strong parsnip taste, incredibly creamy, better mashed with blender
Pumpkin	½ pumpkin	25	Slightly stronger than butternut squash, slightly sweet, smooth
Squash	½ squash	20–25	Mild/bland, slightly sweet, smooth, works well when blended
Swede	1 medium swede	30	Quite mild, a bit astringent, has an aftertaste, tastes good on its own
Sweet potato	3 sweet potatoes	20	Sweet, more texture, less crumbly, orange colour
Turnip	1 large	20–25	Watery, doesn't mash well with a potato masher

All these vegetable mashes can be made, frozen and bagged; they can then be defrosted and added to potato mash to increase the nutrient variety.

CELERIAC MASH

Gluten-free • Grain-free • Dairy-free • Casein-free • Low FODMAP

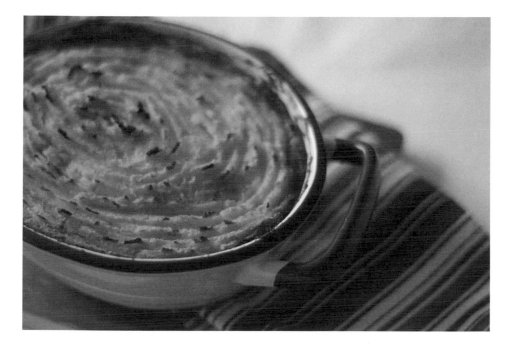

After testing nine types of vegetables (see above), celeriac was near the top of the list. Although it has one of the lowest carbohydrate contents compared to other root vegetables, it has much higher levels of non-starch polysaccharides (a form of fibre that may help to add body to the mash). Celeriac is very difficult to mash, unlike potatoes – so it ideally needs to be blended with a blender. It contains as little as 1.9g of carbohydrate per 100g, and is rich in natural folate. Celeriac is also rich in inorganic nitrate, which helps the cardiovascular system to stay healthy.

1 medium-sized celeriac
Knob of butter

1 Peel the celeriac, and dice into 2.5cm (1 inch) cubes.

2 Boil for 20 minutes, or until tender.

3 Drain the water completely. (Vegetables have a high water content, so no milk is needed for the mash.)

4 Using a hand blender, blend the mixture until smooth.

LASAGNE

Lasagne is a traditional baked pasta dish from Italy. It is traditionally made from flat sheets of cooked pasta with layers of meat, beans or vegetables in tomato sauce covered with a rich cheesy sauce known as béchamel, sprinkled with Parmesan cheese.

In Table 6.2 I have listed examples of replacement options that can be used to help build a more nutritious lasagne dish. For example, instead of using GF pasta sheets you can use thinly sliced courgettes to make the layers. Rather than lean meat you can use lentils, or 50 per cent lean meat and 50 per cent lentils. White sauces can be used as a replacement for tomato-based sauces. The ingredients for this recipe can be taken from the Mince (Ground Meat) and Vegetable Lasagne recipe, Macadamia White Sauce and a choice of GF pasta sheets, eggless pancakes and sliced vegetables.

Table 6.2: Replacement options for the key elements of lasagne

Elements of the lasagne	Replacement options
Pasta sheets	Gluten-free pasta sheets, or homemade pancakes (see Egg-Free Fermented Rice Pancakes recipe) Vegetable sheets such as courgette (zucchini) or butternut squash, thinly sliced
Meat	Lean meat (see Mince (Ground Meat) and Vegetable Lasagne recipe) Legumes Vegetables
Sauce	Homemade tomato sauce, or a creamy sauce if your child cannot tolerate tomato Dairy-free Macadamia White Sauce (see recipe) Ricotta-based sauce Goat's cheese-based sauce

1–2 tbsp olive oil
1 onion
1 carrot
2 cloves garlic
Handful fresh oregano
1 bay leaf
1 portion Mince (Ground Meat) and Vegetable Lasagne (see recipe)

1 Pre-heat oven to 225°C/425°F/gas mark 7.

2 Gently heat 1–2 tbsp of oil in the pan and add onion, carrot and garlic. Season with fresh oregano and a bay leaf and sauté gently for 2–3 minutes.

3 Add various ratios of meat, legumes such as lentils and vegetables such as kale or spinach. (See Mince (Ground Meat) and Vegetable Lasagne recipe to see how to add more vegetables to a meat-based sauce.)

2 portions Macadamia White Sauce (see recipe)

For the layers, 1 portion Egg-Free Fermented Rice Pancakes OR 2 courgettes OR 150g (10 sheets) GF pasta sheets

4 Choose a white sauce, such as the Macadamia White Sauce (prepare double that recipe). Add half of the sauce to the meat/legume/vegetable mixture. Alternatively add 1–2 tbsp of tomato purée.

5 For the layers, thinly slice courgettes, prepare pancakes to use as layers (using the Egg-Free Fermented Rice Pancakes recipe) or prepare GF pasta sheets according to the packet instructions.

6 Spoon half the meat/legume/vegetable/white sauce mixture into the baking dish. Cover the sauce with half of your chosen 'layers'. Spoon half of the remaining white sauce and spread. Repeat process.

7 Bake in oven for 25–30 minutes.

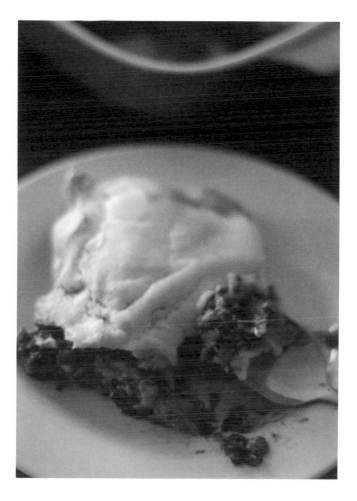

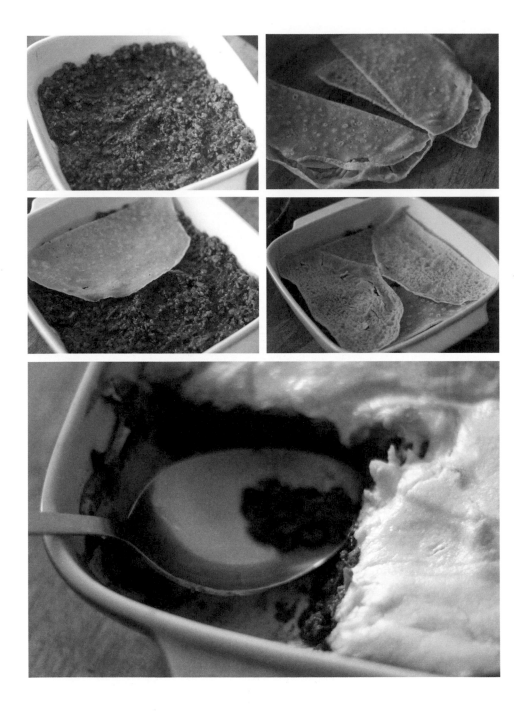

Pasta sheets

You can make vegetable replacements for pasta sheets by thinly slicing courgettes (zucchini) and layering them so that they slightly overlap each other. Add enough courgette slices to cover the tomato-based sauce on each layer, as you would with pasta sheets. Courgettes do not need to be cooked in advance, but they do add a little water to the final dish.

Most other vegetables should be steamed or boiled slightly in advance before adding as layers to the lasagne. I have tried butternut squash, and it works well.

Pancakes can also be used as layers. I think these may be a little easier to digest than the gluten-free lasagne strips for some children. In this recipe I use the Egg-Free Fermented Rice Pancakes recipe from Chapter 5. Once you have cooked them, use them as 'pasta' sheets for the lasagne.

Meat

Lean meats are the best option for lasagne. Also consider using less meat, and replacing some of the meat with vegetables or legumes. These are nutritious and a good source of fibre. Use a 3:2 ratio of meat to vegetables, so about 65 per cent mince (ground meat) and 35 per cent vegetables. You could try some of the following:

- Legumes: fine beans, green beans, split peas, cannellini beans

- Green vegetables: broccoli, kale, lamb's lettuce (yes, it can be cooked!)

- Orange vegetables: butternut squash, sweet potato, pumpkin, carrots

MINCE (GROUND MEAT) AND VEGETABLE LASAGNE

Gluten-free • Grain-free • Dairy-free • Casein-free • SCD • GAPS • Low oxalate •
Low FODMAP

1 medium onion

3-4 tbsp olive oil

1–3 cloves garlic

1 bunch kale (Brussels sprouts or white cabbage, shredded finely, are alternatives for a low phenol option)

300g (1¼ cups) mince (ground meat) – your choice of meat

Pinch of salt

3 tbsp tomato purée (optional)

1 Chop the onion and sauté in 1–2 tbsp olive oil until softened. Add the garlic and sauté for another minute.

2 Add the kale, and cook until tender (about 4 minutes). Season.

3 Process the onion and kale in a food processor, until finely chopped.

4 Stir-fry the mince with 2 tbsp olive oil until cooked.

5 Add the onion, kale and tomato pureé (if using), and cook for 10 minutes.

Sauce
MACADAMIA WHITE SAUCE

Gluten-free • Grain-free • Dairy-free • Casein-free • SCD • GAPS • Low FODMAP

175g (1½ cups) macadamia nuts (or for a low oxalate/phenol option, try cannellini beans)

100ml (½ cup) water

1 clove garlic

Juice of ½ lemon

1 Blend all the ingredients together until smooth.

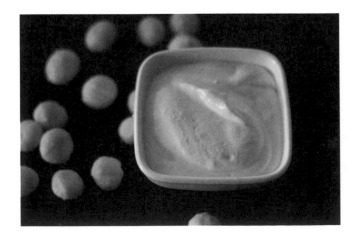

Other Dinner Ideas
SPAGHETTI BOLOGNESE

When making Spaghetti Bolognese, use the same principles as in the Mince (Ground Meat) and Vegetable Lasagne dish above, serving the meat or legumes or vegetables and tomato sauce with spaghetti. You could also replace a little of the spaghetti with spiralized courgette (zucchini) (see page 114).

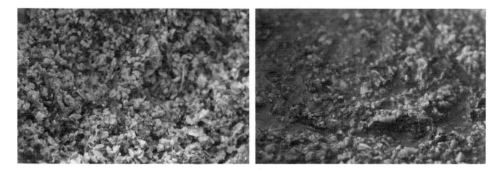

SUPERNOURISHING RICE

Increasing nutrients in a dish is easy when you replace a small portion of a food such as rice with a food that is dense in specific nutrients like carrots. Notice that carrots are a particularly rich source of carotene. Adding a grated carrot to rice would add at least 5360mg of carotene. It would also add at least twice as much fibre. If you do add half a carrot, you may need to cut back on the rice a little – you can always add a little more protein or high-quality fat to make up the difference in calories.

Adding other foods such as 2 teaspoons of almond flour to rice could increase the fibre content by 1.3g. It is easy to see how adding different vegetables, nuts or legumes can increase nutritional density.

There are a few different types of rice that are fibre-rich. These include wild, red, black, wholegrain, brown and white rice. Wild rice has three times more fibre than wholegrain brown rice. White rice has 30 per cent more carbohydrate per gram than wild rice. Substituting wild rice for some white rice could be a good option.

Table 6.3: Nutritional values of Supernourishing Rice

Food name	Qty (g)	Energy (Kcal)	Carb.	Protein	Fat	Fibre	Carotene	Vit. B3	Vit. B5
Carrots, boiled in unsalted water	100	24	4.9	0.6	0.4	2.8	13402	0.1	0.2
Kale, boiled in unsalted water	100	24	1	2.4	1.1	3.5	3375	1.3	0.1
Peas, frozen, boiled in unsalted water	100	69	9.7	6	0.9	7.3	571	2.5	0.1
Butternut squash, baked	100	32	7.4	0.9	0.1	3.2	3255	0.8	0.4
Sweet potato, baked	100	115	28	1.6	0.4	3.1	5140	0.8	0.6
White rice, easy cook, boiled	100	138	31	2.6	1.3	0.8	0	1.5	0.1

Herbs for meat

Research has shown that lemon and herbs can help to cut down the Clostridia count (a common gut bacteria) in meat.[96] Tougher herbs, such as rosemary, sage, oregano and thyme, which have anti-microbial effects, are all good examples. Cumin and cloves have also been found to reduce the Clostridia count in cooked meat. A handful of herbs, such as rosemary or sage, can simply be chopped and added to meat before cooking. Using fresh herbs is preferable to dried.

It's important to buy fresh meat, store it in the fridge and use within three days (though do check the use by date). Most meats need to be cooked thoroughly and served piping hot – check safety guidelines online.

BUTTERNUT SQUASH AND CHICKPEA CURRY

Gluten-free • Grain-free • Dairy-free • Casein-free • Low FODMAP

This recipe is packed full of spices. All of the spices are either known for their antioxidant, anti-inflammatory and/or anti-microbial effects. We have added in butternut squash as this helps to thicken the sauce, alongside the white potato. You can leave out the potato and replace the chickpeas with soaked cannellini beans to make it an SCD dish. If you want it to be lower in phenol, reduce the amount of spices.

½ butternut squash

1 potato (omit for SCD/ GAPS diet)

1 onion

1 tbsp coconut oil

400g (14oz) tin chickpeas (or cannellini beans)

1 tbsp curry powder

Pinch of asafoetida

Pinch of ginger powder

2 pinches of turmeric

Pinch of cumin seeds

Pinch of ground coriander (cilantro)

Pinch of ground cumin

1 tsp Himalayan sea salt

200ml (1 cup) water

1 Chop the butternut squash and potato into small cubes.

2 Slice the onion.

3 Heat 1 tbsp coconut oil or an oil of your choice in a frying pan.

4 Stir-fry the vegetables until the onions are tender (about 3–4 minutes).

5 Add the chickpeas, spices, seasoning and water.

6 Stir and leave to cook for 30 minutes, until the vegetables are tender and the sauce has thickened. White potato is very good at thickening, so if you leave this out, you may need to mash up some of the butternut squash to thicken the sauce.

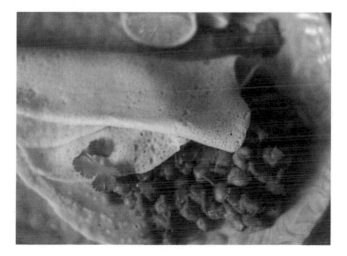

Greens

In Chapters 1 and 2 we spoke about the importance of green vegetables, both as a supply of folate and antioxidants, and as inducers of phase 2 detoxification. The great thing about dietary nutrients is that they come in all shapes and sizes. For example, carotenoids have an orange-red pigment and are packed in foods as families of carotenoids including carotenes, lycopene, xanthophyll, lutein, canthaxanthin, zeaxanthin, violaxanthin, capsorubin and astaxanthin, to name a few. These long-named nutrients stretch in different directions across cell membranes offering antioxidant and anti-inflammatory protection. In Chapter 2, the mitochondria illustration (page 46) shows the different positions of the carotenoids across the cell membrane. The more variety of positions, the better the protection. For this reason, we recommend colourful vegetables.

Dr Joel Fuhrman, in his book *Nutritarian Handbook and ANDI Food Scoring Guide*,[97] created a list of foods that are high in overall nutrient density, giving each food a score. The first 13 ingredients on this superfood list are green leafy vegetables, and are listed in order of nutrient density: kale (cooked), mustard greens, collard greens, turnip greens, watercress, Swiss chard, bok choy, kale (raw), napa cabbage, spinach (cooked), spinach (raw), rocket and green leaf lettuce.

In the recipes below, we show you how to include green vegetables and other vegetables in the diet.

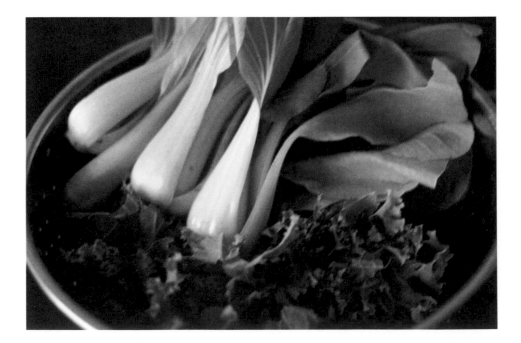

GREEN LEAFY STIR-FRY

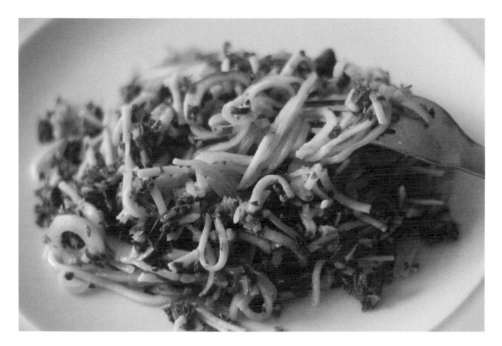

This recipe can be used to add supernourishing greens to noodles.

1 bunch kale

2 medium-sized bok choy

1 onion

Noodles, cooked according to packet instructions

1 Wash the greens.

2 Peel the onion.

3 Finally chop the vegetables in a food processor.

4 Steam for 3–4 minutes.

5 Add the cooked noodles and mix well.

ROCKET PESTO AND PASTA

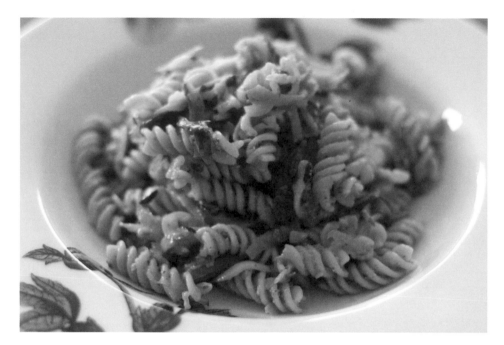

300g (3 cups) gluten-free pasta (4 servings)

15g (¾ cup) rocket

60g (½ cup) macadamia nuts

1 handful basil

1 clove garlic

4 tbsp olive oil

Pinch of salt

1 Cook the pasta in a large pan of boiling water according to the packet instructions.

2 Meanwhile, blend the rest of the ingredients with half of the oil.

3 Add the remaining oil slowly, and pulse through.

4 Mix with the cooked pasta.

LOTS OF VEGETABLES TOMATO SAUCE

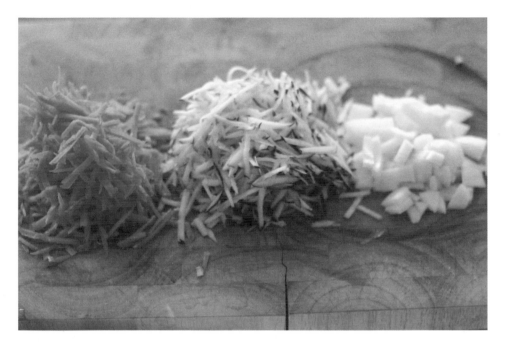

This sauce can be used in any dish requiring tomato sauce.

300g (3 cups) gluten-free pasta (4 servings)

1 carrot

1 courgette (zucchini)

½ onion

1 tbsp olive oil

225g (1 cup) tomato purée

225ml (1 cup) water

1 Cook the pasta in a large pan of boiling water according to the packet instructions.

2 Grate the carrot and courgette and peel and slice the onion.

3 Add the olive oil to a wok and stir-fry the vegetables for 3–4 minutes.

4 Blend the vegetables with a hand blender.

5 Add the tomato purée with a little water.

6 Add to the cooked pasta and serve.

7 Snacks

Snacking is defined as a small amount of food eaten in-between meals. Grazing can be seen as constant or unregulated snacking. Many snacks tend to be quite processed and are usually high in carbohydrates. As digestive enzymes are released following a daily rhythm synchronized with food,[98] if we snack all day or eat food irregularly, this can put a strain on the digestive processes.

If there is small intestine bacterial overgrowth, constant snacking may lead to extra 'food' for bacteria and promote a greater imbalance in the gut community. Even dentists talk about the importance of regularity, because constant grazing exposes the teeth to food throughout the day, and carbohydrate-rich food combined with oral bacteria increases oral pH, which increases the risk of dental caries.[99]

Regular mealtimes are also important as blood sugar regulation has a big effect on many behaviours in children. This can be exaggerated in a child with autism, as they can become hypoglycemic, which more rapidly leads to challenging behaviours.

Ideally, regular meal and snack times are recommended, without any grazing or snacking. This may be a challenge at first, and you may need to begin with a gradual reduction of access to foods throughout the day.

I have found that if the diet is improved first by reducing sugars and increasing lower GI foods, the transition is easier from constant grazing to regular snack times. I have also questioned whether imbalances in gut flora drive some of these grazing behaviours.

Consistency in this process is key so that children can get into healthier habits. Inconsistency (e.g. if sometimes the children are allowed to graze continually and at other times they are not) could lead to tantrums. A bit of extra work and discipline will be required at first.

The recipes included in this section are aimed at providing two types of snacks. The first is a lower GI snack; the second is a blended snack in the form of an ice pop or smoothie (see Chapter 8 for more options). The reasoning behind this is that if the food is already blended (mechanically broken down), it can be more easily digested, so there is less 'food' lying around for microbes between meals.

Some of these choices do contain sugar, but they are less processed and lower in GI than shop-bought snacks.

HONEY ALMOND SQUARES

Gluten-free • Grain-free • Dairy-free • Casein-free • SCD • GAPS • Low FODMAP

450g (2 cups) blanched almond flour

¼ tsp sea salt

¼ tsp baking soda

¼ cup manuka honey

1 tbsp vanilla extract

1 Mix the flour, salt and baking soda in one bowl.

2 Mix the oil, honey and vanilla extract in another bowl.

3 Combine the two bowls of ingredients together well.

4 Place in the fridge for at least 1 hour.

5 Preheat the oven to 165ºC/325ºF/gas mark 3.

6 Roll the mixture out between two sheets of parchment paper, until about 1.2cm (½ inch) thick.

7 Cut into fingers and pierce with a fork.

8 Bake for 10 minutes.

9 Leave to cool on a cooling rack.

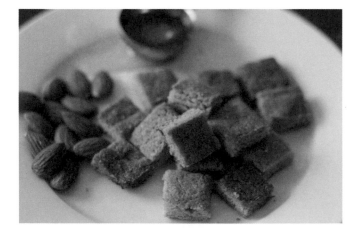

AKARA

Gluten-free • Grain-free • Dairy-free • Casein-free • SCD • GAPS • Low phenol •
Low oxalate • Low FODMAP

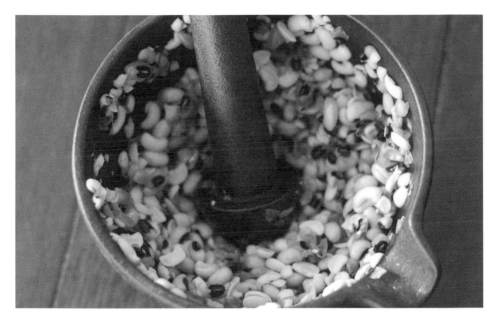

180g (1 cup) black-eyed beans

1 spring onion (scallion)

Pinch of salt

½ saucepan of rice bran oil

1 Soak the black-eyed beans for two days, changing the water regularly.

2 Using a pestle and mortar, grind the beans to lose some of their skins.

3 Rinse off some of the skins, but don't worry if you can't remove them all.

4 Using a food processor or a hand blender, grind the beans until they reach a thick consistency. Do not over-blend.

5 Chop the spring onion and add it to the food-processed mixture.

6 Half-fill a saucepan with rice bran oil and bring it to a medium heat.

7 Using an ice-cream scoop or tablespoon, scoop out the mixture and carefully add the scoops to the heated oil, one by one. Deep fry them for a few minutes, until they are golden brown and cooked inside. (Note: If the oil is too hot the akaras will burn, or they'll go brown before they're cooked inside.)

SUNFLOWER SEED BUTTER ICE POPS

Gluten-free • Grain-free • Dairy-free • Casein-free • SCD • GAPS • Low phenol • Low oxalate • Low FODMAP

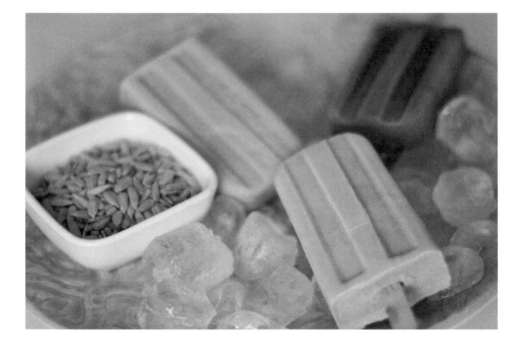

Nut ingredients and ice pops are a wonderful combination, partly because of the high fat content of nuts, which lends itself well to the creamy texture needed for ice cream or ice pops. These ice pops have a low GI and are packed with calories. You could also make liquid snacks for children who like to graze all day, as they are easier for the body to digest than, for example, a constant supply of rice cakes. As these ice pops are seed-based, they can be an option for those with a nut allergy who can tolerate seeds, and those who are on a lower oxalate diet. The Himalayan salt in this recipe is thought to be richer in minerals than table salt, and the coconut oil helps to make the mixture smooth.

400ml (1¾ cup) coconut milk

3 tbsp sunflower seed butter

60ml (¼ cup) agave syrup (or ½ tsp stevia)

1 banana (optional)

Pinch of Himalayan salt

1 tbsp coconut oil (optional)

1 Combine all the ingredients in a blender.

2 Freeze in ice pop moulds.

CAULIFLOWER POPCORN

Gluten-free • Grain-free • Dairy-free • Casein-free • SCD • GAPS • Low oxalate •
High polyol FODMAP

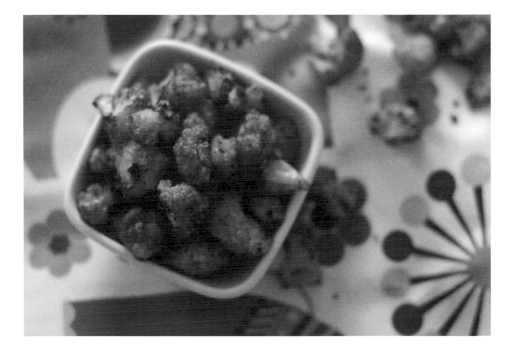

1 head of cauliflower

1 tbsp olive oil, or oil of your choice

1 tsp mild paprika

1 Heat the oven to 210°C/425°F/gas mark 7.

2 Break the cauliflower into small florets.

3 Add the oil to the cauliflower with the paprika. Mix with your hands (this is a child-friendly job, though if the child has sensitive skin you may want to do this for them).

4 Place on a greaseproof oven tray and bake for 10 minutes, or until golden.

TWIGS

Gluten-free • Dairy-free • Casein-free • Low FODMAP

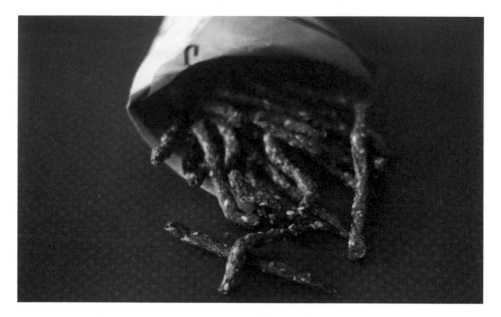

180g (1 cup) quinoa

180g (1 cup) short-grain brown rice

2 tsp tamari

⅓ cup flax seeds

2 tsp sea salt

1 Cook the quinoa and rice together according to the packet instructions.

2 Once the quinoa and rice are cooked, blend with a hand blender until smooth.

3 Add in all the remaining ingredients and blend together.

4 Using a piping bag, pipe the mixture into short strips.

5 Preheat the oven to 180°C/350°F/gas mark 4.

6 Bake for 10–12 minutes. Leave to cool before serving.

COURGETTE (ZUCCHINI) CHIPS

Gluten-free • Grain-free • Dairy-free • Casein-free • SCD • GAPS • Low phenol (peel the courgette) • Low oxalate • Low FODMAP

1 large courgette (zucchini)

2 tbsp olive oil

Pinch of sea salt

1 Slice the courgette thinly, using a knife or mandolin.

2 Dehydrate at 125°C/260°F/gas mark ½ in a dehydrator for 8 hours. Alternatively bake in the oven at 150°C/200°F/gas mark 2 for 2–3 hours. (Note the time needed varies according to the type of oven used.)

SUPER-SIMPLE OAT COOKIES

Gluten-free • Dairy-free • Casein-free • Low oxalate (moderate, banana) • Low FODMAP

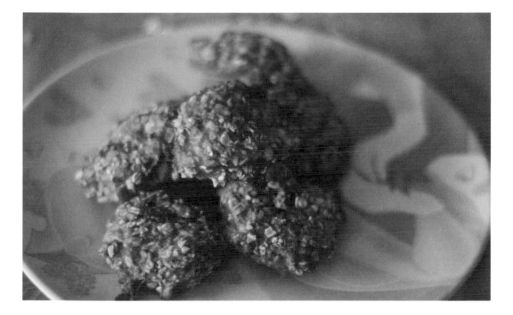

2 large ripe bananas
150g (1 cup) rolled oats

1 Preheat the oven to 180ºC/350ºF/gas mark 4.

2 Mash the bananas with a fork.

3 Mix in the oats.

4 Using a tablespoon, drop the mixture onto a baking tray lined with baking paper.

5 Bake for 15 minutes.

MUESLI CRACKERS

Gluten-free • Dairy-free • Casein-free • Low FODMAP

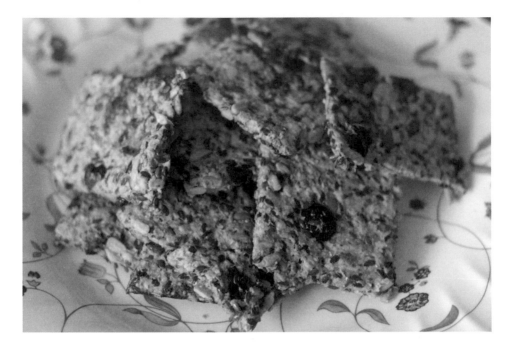

This makes two baking sheets of crackers.

70g (½ cup) sunflower seeds

50g (¼ cup) flax seeds

2 tbsp pumpkin seeds

1 tbsp sesame seeds

150g (¾ cup) rolled oats

1 tbsp desiccated coconut

1 tbsp chia seeds

2 tbsp psyllium seed husks (3 tbsp if using psyllium husk powder)

½ tsp fine grain sea salt

1½ tbsp coconut oil, melted

350g (1½ cups) water

1 Preheat the oven to 180ºC/350ºF/gas mark 4.

2 Combine all the ingredients and leave to rest for two hours.

3 Place between 2 sheets of parchment paper, and firmly roll out until flat.

4 Score gently with a knife.

5 Peel off the top layer of parchment paper, and place the mixture together with the bottom layer of parchment paper on a baking tray.

6 Bake for 20 minutes.

7 Turn the crackers over and bake for a further 10 minutes.

8 Leave to cool.

BREADSTICKS

Gluten-free • Grain-free • Dairy-free • Casein-free • SCD • GAPS • Low FODMAP

170g (1½ cups) almond flour

1 egg

2 tsp extra virgin oil

¼ tsp salt

¼ tsp baking soda

1 Preheat oven to 350ºC/180ºF/gas mark 4.

2 Beat the egg in a bowl, then add remaining ingredients to the egg.

3 Divide the dough into eight equal parts and roll out to create finger-thick breadsticks.

4 Place on a parchment paper lined baking tray and bake for 15 minutes.

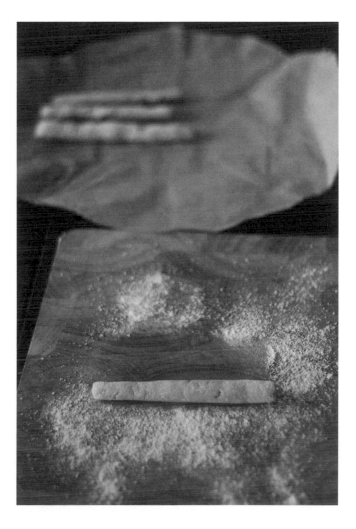

8 Drinks

Drinking habits vary between children. Some avoid water completely, only drinking fruit cordials and juices, while others drink one cup of water after another. Still others prefer not to drink fluids because of discomfort or pain, or other sensory-based issues. Not drinking enough fluid can lead to mild dehydration, and the big challenge is that many children with autism may feel thirsty but may not ask for a drink. This means planning regular water/fluid intake to ensure they stay hydrated.

Water is so important that even a 1 per cent reduction in the body alerts it to start rehydrating. Proper hydration is needed for optimum function of the whole brain and body. Our DNA (genetic material) tells the body how to work through communicating via proteins (a process known as DNA expression), and even this can be affected by poor hydration. Dehydration can also lead to impaired mental function including problems with concentration, motivation and alertness, and it can increase irritability. Symptoms such as headaches, constipation and fatigue can be caused or worsened by dehydration.[100]

Table 8.1: Symptoms and signs that may
be observed with dehydration[101]

Function	Symptoms	Signs
Cognitive	Impaired concentration Impaired short-term memory Reduced alertness Increased perceived effort Reduced motivation Irritability	
Urine and bowel movements		Dark urine (appearance should be straw-coloured) Decreased urine volume Constipation (<3 bowel movements/week)
Additional symptoms	Headache Lightheadedness Fatigue Sunken eyes Dry skin	Lack of tear production Dry skin

Children are more vulnerable to dehydration than adults. Children have a higher metabolic rate, and their kidneys do not conserve water as well as adults; in addition, they lose more water from their skin through breathing. Because conserving water uses up lots of energy, dehydration can cause unnecessary stress to the kidneys (oxidative stress).

Dehydration can also increase the risk of urinary tract infections. About 1 per cent of boys and 3 per cent of girls experience urinary tract infections in the first ten years of life.

There are recommended guidelines for water intake for babies, children and adults (see Table 8.2).

According to studies, people in the US and UK take in about 20 per cent of their water from food. Food varies in water content. Table 8.3 gives an idea of the percentage of water content contained in a sample of foods. Fruits and vegetables tend to have a higher water content than higher-protein foods or bread.

Table 8.2: Recommended fluid intake, by age[102]

Age	Recommended fluid intake	250ml (glass/cup) average of water or other beverage
0–6 months	100–190ml/day	–
6–12 months	800–1000ml/day	–
2 years	1110–1200ml/day	3.5–4.5 cups
2–3 years	1300ml/day	4–5 cups
4–8 years	1600ml/day	5–6.5 cups
9–13 years	2100ml/day	7–8.5 cups
14+ years	2000ml (female) 2500ml (male)	6.5–8 cups 8–10 cups

Table 8.3: Percentage of water content in a selection of foods

% of water content	Foods
100	Water
90–99	Melons, strawberries, lettuce, cabbage, celery, spinach, squash (cooked)
80–89	Fruit juice, yoghurt, apples, grapes, oranges, carrots, broccoli (cooked), pears, pineapple
70–79	Bananas, avocado, ricotta cheese, potato (baked), corn (cooked)
60–69	Pasta, legumes, salmon, ice cream, chicken breast
50–59	Mince (ground beef), hot dogs, feta cheese
40–49	Pizza
30–39	Bagels, bread
20–29	Cakes, biscuits
10–19	Butter, margarine, dried fruits
1–9	Walnuts, peanuts, cookies, cereals, nut butters
0	Oils and sugars

We need to plan how to ensure fluids are available to children, especially if the child is non-verbal, has language delays, or any impairment that might influence their ability to ask for water or drinks.

Access to water at school and when children are away from home is also important. Research suggests that up to 71 per cent of children in school may not drink sufficient water to maintain hydration. This can be detrimental, as dehydration affects academic performance.

If sufficient water is drunk during the day, a child of six may be visiting the toilet about six to seven times daily. This has to be planned into the school day or at home.

Extra special attention to fluid intake should be given to children who are ill with the flu or other infections, when they have a temperature, or have been vomiting or have diarrhoea, as dehydration can occur more rapidly. It is also important to consider sufficient water intake in hotter weather and when children are exercising. The following box suggests ways you can increase your child's fluid intake.

Methods for increasing fluid and water intake

- A water bottle – provide a water bottle for your child and have it available for your child in the room where they are.

- Ice is another form of fluid intake, and some children with hyposensitivity enjoy crunching it.

- Soups are another way of getting in more fluid, but consider that it may reduce the overall calorific intake of the meal.

- Juices are considered by many in the 'juicing community' to provide 'structured' water that is considered to be more hydrating.

- Smoothies are another way of increasing fluid intake.

- Ice pops can be another form of increasing fluid intake.

- Fruit and vegetables generally have a higher water content, so these can be increased in the diet.

- Dilute fruit juices with 25–75 per cent water over time, or more gradually if your child is particularly sensitive to taste changes.

You may want to introduce one new method of increasing fluid intake at a time. Ideally, we want children to drink more water rather than other fluids or food with a high water content, so thinking of ways of helping your child drink more pure water is important. Below are some ideas of how to increase fluid intake overall. You may need to try some of these new ways of fluid intake a few times, and may even need assistance from an ABA therapist. Each child is different, so see what method seems to work for your child.

Water, Juices, Smoothies, Teas and Ices

We now consider water, juices, smoothies, teas and ices as ways of increasing water and fluid content. We look at the pros and cons of different types of water. We then look at juices and how to juice, with practical suggestions for preparing fruits, vegetables, herbs and spices and sprouts for juicing, as well as considering the ingredients in juices within the context of food sensitivities. The basics of building a smoothie are explored, and recipes for herbal teas, waters and ices are given.

Water

'Water is not present simply to fill up the available space in and around biological proteins.'[103] A certain amount of water is needed for the biological activity of all proteins. Most soluble enzymes require a substantial amount of water to work. Even DNA requires a certain amount of hydration to coil up or unravel.

Water in nature is not chemically pure H_2O. It contains small amounts of gases, minerals and organic matter. Minerals in water are present in their ionic form, meaning that they are electrically charged. In this form they are easily absorbed by the digestive tract. Mineral levels in water vary considerably depending on the source and processing of the water.

There are many different types of water available.

Table 8.4: Different types of water

Type of water	Pros	Cons
Tap.	A source of minerals such as calcium, magnesium, sodium, potassium, iron, copper, zinc and manganese. These are available naturally or added during the processing of drinking water.	Can have disinfectant residues used in water-cleansing process.
Well water, sourced from groundwater in aquifers, usually drawn by a pump. The water sourced varies in quality.	Increased protection from surface contaminants and bacteria.	Concentrations of arsenic are higher than in tap water.
Spring water, rising from the earth's surface from an underground aquifer. It is collected from a natural source, but unlike mineral water, can be processed to remove excess grit and dirt.		Can be contaminated if close to non-organic farm land.
Filtered water.	Filtering helps to remove chlorine, chemicals, herbicides and pesticides. Carbon filters can also remove odours, tastes and colour.	Trace minerals remain. Filtering does not effectively remove microorganisms. The filter needs replacing regularly due to build-up of contaminants.
Distilled water, vaporized using a heat source. The vaporized water then goes into a condenser, where the water is cooled and returns to liquid.	Distillation removes bacteria and some viruses and heavy metals such as lead, arsenic and mercury.	Pesticides, herbicides and synthetic chemicals are not removed in the process. Distillation strips water of natural trace minerals. The dietary intake of toxic metals is increased. Directly affects intestinal mucous membrane, metabolism and mineral balance.[104]

Reverse osmosis, where the water has been passed through a membrane with tiny pores that can fit molecules the same size as a water molecule. Bigger molecules such as lead, chlorine and other heavy metals as well as minerals are removed.	Removes bacteria, larger viruses and larger molecules.	Removes natural minerals. Membranes can become blocked or damaged. Some reverse osmosis membranes can be damaged by chlorine. Pesticides, herbicides and chlorine may be able to pass through the membrane.
Soft water has a higher concentration of sodium ions. It can occur naturally or water can be treated with sodium to reduce calcium and magnesium.	Soft water is not considered to be healthy to drink.	It is thought to dissolve metals such as cadmium and lead from pipes more easily.
Hard water contains minerals measured by the amount of calcium and magnesium ions.	Some studies suggest a reduced risk of specific concerns.[105]	Increased risk of cardiovascular disease with increased water hardness.
Sparkling water, bottled water that has natural carbonation or carbonation through highly pressurized carbon dioxide gas.	Some children enjoy fizzy drinks, and at first fizzy water can be used to dilute fizzy drinks, or be added to juices to help reduce the sugar/fructose content of the drink or juice.	Carbonated water can impact health as it contains high levels of phosphates. Phosphorus can leach calcium from the bones and can lead to a higher risk of osteoporosis if consumed excessively.

Juices

In clinic I find that many children enjoy cordials, fruit juice drinks, coconut water and fruit juice. On the healthier side, many parents juice fresh fruit and vegetables for their children. It goes without saying that not all juice is equal. Added sugars, pasteurization, preservatives, flavours and colours can all have an effect on the flavour, nutrient density and potential reactions that children have when they drink juice. Certain tiny substances such as oxalates and salicylates can be concentrated in fruit juices. These can influence symptoms and behaviour in children who are sensitive to these substances. Others react to the small sugars such as high levels of fructose or polyols (alcohol sugars). I have seen children improve just by cutting out shop-bought juices from their diet.

One of the benefits of homemade juice is that it is another way to get fruits and vegetables into the child, as well as being high in water content for hydration. Some children who would never touch a green vegetable will eat Green Juice Lollies freely.

There is often confusion about the difference between blending and juicing. Juicing is the removal of pulp from the juice, and blending pulverizes the whole fruit or vegetable. Removal of pulp in juicing significantly reduces fibre content.

Table 8.5: Comparing the nutritional content of orange juice to an orange

Nutrients and GI/GL	1 glass (250ml) orange juice	1 medium orange
Energy (kcal)	83	59
Carbohydrate	20	13.6
Protein	1.5	1.8
Fibre	0.3	2.9
Sugar	20	13.6
Glucose	5	3.5
Fructose	5.5	3.8
Sucrose	10	6.2
Vitamin C	120	86
GI (estimated)	115	67
GL	9.2	4.6

Glycaemic Load

Glycaemic load takes into account the quantity or portion of the food that is to raise blood sugar levels using the glycaemic index ranking system.

Table 8.5 shows how the carbohydrate content is at least 30 per cent greater in the orange juice than in the orange. There is also a 90 per cent fibre reduction. However, the remaining 10 per cent of fibre still contains soluble fibres such as pectins, gums and mucilages.

Juicing is generally a supernourishing technique where you can concentrate plant nutrients by removing fibre. It also maximizes nutrient intake as juice is easy to digest. For example, drinking juice increases beta-carotene levels more than eating whole fruits.[106] This is not to say that it is better to drink juice than to eat whole fruit, just that juicing can be a method we can use to increase the concentration of nutrients. In addition, some children have challenges processing fibre, and juices are easier on their system.

There are several concerns about juicing that are worth discussing, however. The first is that when a fruit or vegetable is juiced, there is a rise in the GI. Children who become irritable or who have melt-downs when hungry may respond better to vegetable than fruit juices, as vegetable juices usually have less sugar and a lower GI.

There is also the issue of yeast overgrowth. Juicing fruit can increase both sucrose or fructose levels by three to four times in comparison with the whole fruit. So again, juicing vegetables may be recommended for those children who respond negatively to high fructose.

Another concern is that the level of pesticides sprayed on fruit and vegetables can become concentrated in fruit juice. The list below (see Table 8.6) is taken from the Environmental Health Working Group 2014. It lists 12 fruits that have the highest pesticide residue from the foods sampled (the dirty dozen). The 'clean 15' are the fruits and vegetables that had the lowest levels of pesticide residues in the foods sampled. If using fruit and vegetables from the dirty dozen list, it is best to soak them in a bowl with some grapeseed extract. Research suggests that this helps to remove some of the residues.[107] Alternatively, rinse them thoroughly in water.

Table 8.6: The 'dirty dozen' and the 'clean 15'

Dirty dozen	Clean 15
Apples	Avocado
Strawberries	Sweetcorn
Grapes	Pineapple
Celery	Cabbage
Peaches	Garden peas, frozen
Spinach	Onions
Sweet peppers	Asparagus
Nectarines	Mango
Cucumbers	Papaya
Cherry tomatoes	Kiwi
Sugar snap peas	Aubergine (eggplant)
Potatoes	Grapefruit
	Cantaloupe melon
	Cauliflower
	Sweet potato

Below are some guidelines for juicing.

- Always wash or peel produce. You can soak the vegetables or fruit in Veggie Wash®, lemon juice or a few drops of grapeseed extract to help to reduce any pesticide residues. Peel non-organic produce.

- Buy organic where possible, especially if the foods fall into the dirty dozen category.

- Peel oranges, tangerines and grapefruits as the skin contains volatile oils that can cause digestive problems in some people. Leave the pithy part as that is full of vitamin C and bioflavonoids (vitamins that act as antioxidants).

- Peel mangoes and papaya as their skins contain oils that can cause skin irritation.

- Remove pits, stones and seeds from peaches, nectarines, plums, apricots, cherries and mangoes.

- Remove seeds from papaya as these are hot.

- Bananas, berries, avocado and other soft fruit do not juice well. It is best to juice watery fruits in the juicer. Add the juice and soft fruit to the blender to make a mixed smoothie-type juice.

- Light, air and heat can all lead to nutrient loss. The juice turns brown or becomes discoloured once oxidized.

- Slow masticating juicers seem to allow the juice to last longer.

- Pulp can be used in soups, muffins or as compost.

Table 8.7: Base fruits and vegetables for juices

	Fruit and vegetables	Additional comments
Base	Carrot, sweet potato, cucumber, celery, beetroot, orange, apple	Carrot (moderate oxalate) Sweet potato, cucumber, celery, beetroot (high oxalate) Orange, apple (high fructose, not tolerated by some children)
Leafy vegetables	Lettuce, kale, spinach, Swiss chard	Kale (high phenol/salicylate) Spinach (high oxalate) Swiss chard (high oxalate)
Bitter greens	Rocket, endive, kale, sorrel, tatsoi, watercress, mustard greens, frisée, radish	Rocket, kale, sorrel, watercress (all high phenol)
Root vegetables	Beetroot, carrot, parsnip, turnip	Beetroot (oxalate)
Texture	Banana, papaya, berries, avocado	Berries (high phenol) Avocado (high salicylate)
Flavour	Ginger, turmeric, herbs (mint, coriander (cilantro), parsley), chilli, lime, lemons, garlic, strawberry	Ginger, turmeric (high salicylates)
Low fructose	Granny Smith apples, lemon, cranberries, blackberries, blackcurrants, raspberries, strawberries	Berries (high salicylate/high phenol) Granny Smith apples (high salicylate)
Exotic	Mango, pineapple, passion fruit, kiwi	Pineapple (high sucrose) Kiwi (high salicylate) Passion fruit (moderate salicylate)

You can choose to use one vegetable when juicing, such as carrots, to give 100 per cent carrot juice, or you can mix a selection of fruits or vegetables to create a mixed juice. When creating a mixed juice, there are a few things to consider. The first is the idea of selecting a base fruit or vegetable. This would be a fruit or vegetable that yields a large quantity of juice. You can then select a range of fruits or vegetables as add-ons that can be used to increase the nutritional density of the juice, such as green leafy vegetables, or you could add texture, such as bananas, or extra flavour, such as ginger.

Juice can be frozen into ice, and one of the good things about doing this is that it tends to blunt the flavour of a food, so the flavour of stronger-tasting fruits or vegetables can be slightly masked. As ice can be a sensory-seeking choice for some children, it can be another way to get fruit and vegetable juices into the child's diet.

Smoothies

A smoothie is a blended drink. Choose something watery as a base, such as milk, water, coconut water or juice. Then add in additional foods for texture or flavour, such as strawberry for flavour and banana for texture. In addition, you can add superfoods such as lucuma (lucuma comes from the lucuma fruit, which grows high in the mountains of Peru and can be bought as a powder). One of the benefits of smoothies is that the foods are thoroughly blended, with their skin (including fibre) broken down. This can help those who do not chew properly when eating. They can also be used to increase calorific intake (especially with the addition of protein powders or other ingredients such as lucuma or coconut oil/oils/fats, as these have high calorific values). Smoothies can also be used between meals as a liquid snack to support blood sugar regulation, especially if proteins or fats are added to improve glycaemic control.

Smoothies can also be turned into ice lollies. Some children who would not drink a smoothie will eat an ice lolly, and these can also be used as a replacement for snacks.

Building a smoothie

BASE: Add a watery base

Water

Coconut water (high electrolyte rehydrating/naturally sweet – no need to add sweetener)

Juice (can choose from juicing options – the juice can come fresh from the juicer)

Nut/seed milk (home-made is best for the good-quality fats, but some nuts are high in oxalates or phenols or are just difficult to digest due to fibres and high fat)

Cereal-based milks

Soy-based milks (soy is highly allergenic, in the top 8 allergenic foods)

Blended nuts or seeds (low GI)

Water and protein powder (various types of protein powders – rice, pea, hemp, soya, whey; low GI)

If your child likes ice you can add 4 ice cubes.

FLAVOURS AND TEXTURE:

These can be added fresh or frozen. If frozen you will get an icier, thicker consistency

Berries (phenols, salicylates)

Banana (high fructose and sucrose – ripe bananas can be used)

Avocado (high salicylate, low GI)

Kale (high phenol, low GI)

Rocket (high phenol, low GI)

Pear (salicylate)

EXTRA FIBRE:

Chia seeds (high salicylate, low GI)

Flaxseed (high salicylate, low GI)

Oats (low GI)

Herbs and Spices in Teas and Drinks

Culinary herbs are packed with nutrients. For example, parsley contains about 100 times more phenolic compounds compared to the same weight of kale. Herbs can be used to make herb waters, where the herb is passed through the juicer and then water is added. Or hot water can be added to culinary herbs and left to infuse. This can then be used as a base for smoothies, as ice cubes, or as a hot drink.

Table 8.8: Different herbs and spices for use in teas

Herbs	Spices
Parsley, thyme, marjoram, lemongrass, lemon verbena, rosemary, dill, sage, tarragon, chives, basil, oregano	Ginger, turmeric, cardamom, cinnamon

Teas
SAGE TEA

Gluten-free • Grain-free • Dairy-free • Casein-free • SCD • GAPS • Low oxalate • Low FODMAP

8–10 fresh sage leaves

250–300ml (1–1¼ cups) water

1 Cover the sage leaves with freshly boiled water.

2 Leave to steep for 10 minutes.

3 Drink or freeze.

TURMERIC AND LEMON TEA

Gluten-free • Grain-free • Dairy-free • Casein-free • SCD • GAPS • Low FODMAP

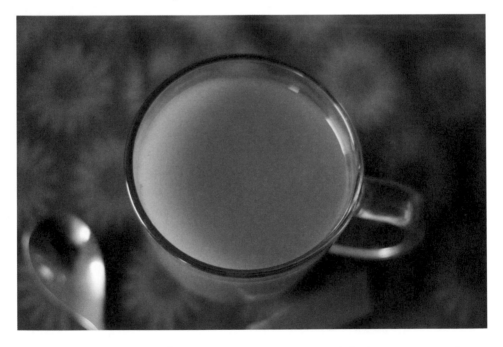

2 tbsp fresh turmeric, grated

Juice of 1 lemon

750ml (3 cups) hot water

1 Add the grated turmeric and the lemon juice to the hot water and leave to steep for 20 minutes.

Lemonades
NO-SUGAR LEMONADE

Gluten-free • Grain-free • Dairy-free • Casein-free • SCD • GAPS • Low oxalate •
Low FODMAP

This can also be used to make ice pops – just add in a little extra stevia or xylitol
to sweeten.

3 fresh lemons

½ tsp stevia (moderate
oxalate) or xylitol (low
oxalate)

900ml (4 cups) naturally
carbonated or still water

1 Slice the lemons in half, and using a citrus juicer or a
fork, squeeze the juice into a jug, removing any seeds.

2 Add the stevia or xylitol, and stir.

3 Add the water and stir.

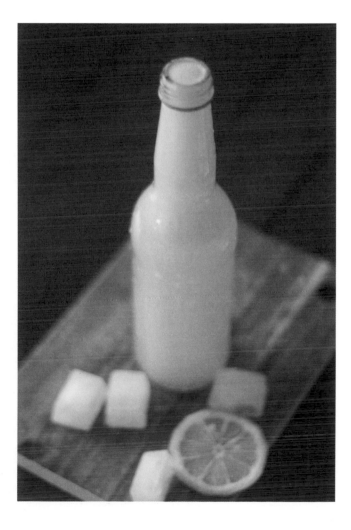

PINEAPPLE LEMONADE

Gluten-free • Grain-free • Dairy-free • Casein-free • SCD • GAPS • Low phenol • Low oxalate • Low FODMAP

Pineapple has a high level of sucrose (a natural fruit sugar), but is low in fructose. The sucrose makes it particularly sweet when the fruit is ripe. To test for ripeness, try pulling out one of the leaves from the pineapple – it should come out easily. The pineapple will sweeten the sour lemon, which is also a low fructose fruit.

1 pineapple

3 lemons

300ml (1¼ cup) sparkling water

Ice

1 Juice the pineapple and lemons.

2 Combine in a jug with the sparkling water and ice.

GREEN LEMONADE

Gluten-free • Grain-free • Dairy-free • Casein-free • SCD • GAPS • Low oxalate • Low FODMAP

2 green apples

1 handful kale

1 lemon

¼ thumb of ginger

1 Juice all the ingredients together.

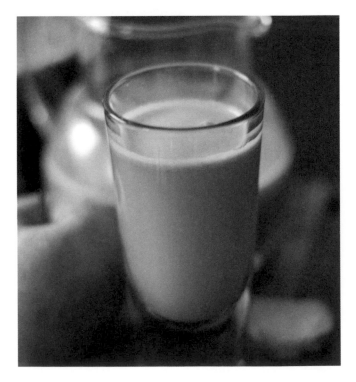

Ice Lollies
BASIL ICE POPS

Gluten-free • Grain-free • Dairy-free • Casein-free • SCD • GAPS • Low FODMAP

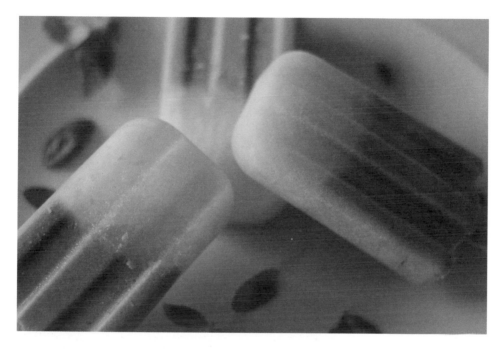

10 basil leaves

120ml (½ cup) lime juice

¼ cup coconut oil

½ cup water

1 Blend all the ingredients together.

2 Pour into ice lolly containers and freeze.

GREEN JUICE LOLLY

Gluten-free • Grain-free • Dairy-free • Casein-free • SCD • GAPS • Low phenol • Low oxalate • Low FODMAP

1 cucumber (very low oxalate)

3 outer romaine lettuce leaves (very low oxalate)

2 Granny Smith apples (low oxalate)

1 lemon (low oxalate)

1 Juice all the ingredients together.

2 Freeze.

Juices
ANTI-INFLAMMATORY ORANGE JUICE

Gluten-free • Grain-free • Dairy-free • Casein-free • SCD • GAPS • Low oxalate (moderate) • Low FODMAP

1 thumb of fresh turmeric, peeled

½ thumb of fresh ginger, peeled

2–3 carrots, juiced

1 orange, juiced

1 papaya, peeled and seeds removed

1 Juice the turmeric, ginger, carrots and orange.

2 Blend with the papaya.

ZINGY CARROT AND APPLE JUICE

Gluten-free • Grain-free • Dairy-free • Casein-free • SCD • GAPS • Low oxalate (moderate) • Low FODMAP

3 carrots

2 apples

1 thumb of ginger

1 Juice all the ingredients together.

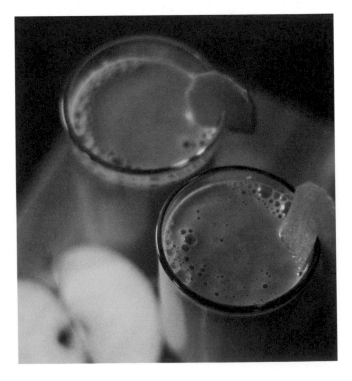

GARDEN FRUIT JUICE

Gluten-free • Grain-free • Dairy-free • Casein-free • SCD • GAPS • Low phenol •
Low oxalate • Low FODMAP

2 oranges

2 apples

6 big romaine lettuce
leaves

1 Juice all the ingredients together.

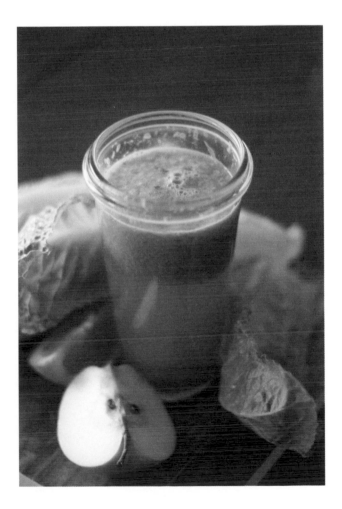

DARK GREEN PEAR JUICE

Gluten-free • Grain-free • Dairy-free • Casein-free • SCD • GAPS • Low FODMAP

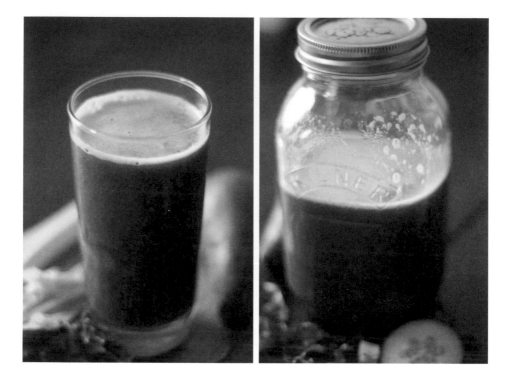

1 cucumber

3 sticks of celery

1 pear

3 handfuls of kale

1 Juice all the ingredients together.

It may take time for your child to try a new juice, smoothie or tea, but do not give up. Keep introducing different types of healthier drinks at home, school or when they are away from home, and see what types of drinks they like. Maybe offer slight varieties of these drinks to help increase nutrient and fluid intake.

PART III

MEAL CHOICE AND TRANSITIONING TO HEALTHIER FOODS

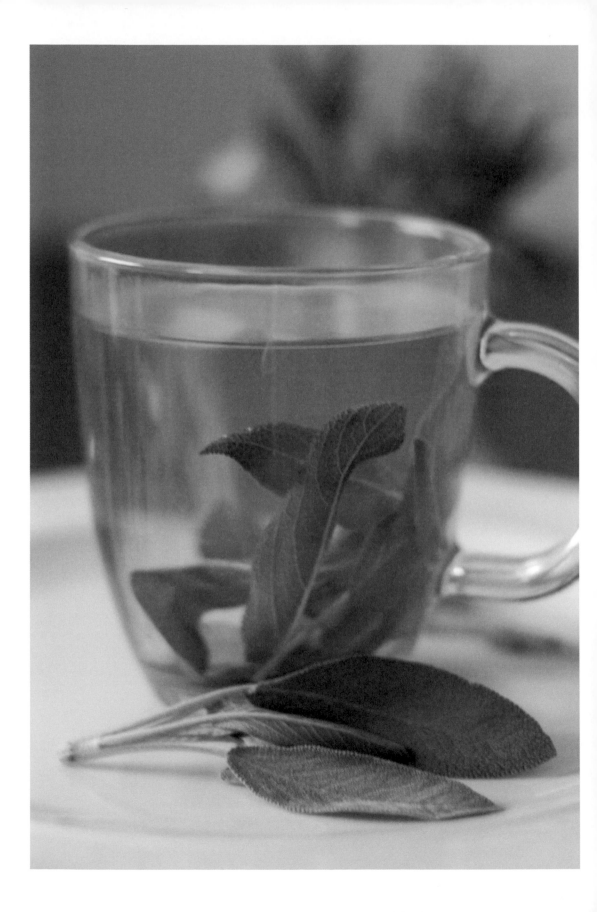

9 Top Tips for Menu Planning and Meal Building

How to Plan a Menu

Menu planning can be quite a challenge when you need to cook different things for different family members. Deciding what to eat, buy, cook and serve as a meal is one of the biggest challenges families can face. Many parents give up because they feel overwhelmed with the enormity of the task. It is for this reason that menu planning is based on a system of replacing foods. That way parents can choose what they can manage, and over the weeks they can introduce more dietary changes.

Some of the keys to change are to start small, keep it simple, and keep going – planning and consistency. Decide on a menu, write a plan and practise, practise, practise. Just like learning to play a piano, you practise and practise until your new skill (or dietary change) becomes natural to you. When we are learning to play the piano and we make a mistake, we don't think we might as well give up because we have made a mistake; instead we just recognize that we need more practice.

You also need to be honest with yourself. Are you really going to get up 30 minutes earlier to prepare breakfast? Or should you prepare it the night before? Are you really going to try five new recipes a week? Or is one recipe a month more realistic? The more successful you are at achieving your goals, the more likely it is that you will feel confident and can build in more goals towards success.

The brain and the body are designed to create habits that increase our efficiency. So one of the reasons why old habits die hard is because the brain is trying to hold onto the old ways. Replacing an old habit with a new habit is one of the ways that you can rewire your brain, so that although the old habit is trying to 'fire', the new habit crowds it out. Eventually, the new habit will become easier, but it is usually a lot of hard work in the beginning. And this is why planning is helpful, because it focuses the mind on the goal.

The first question to ask in the menu planning process is, as I have said before, clear evaluation of where you are now, which is fundamental to any change. If you spend five minutes preparing breakfast now, how can the diet be modified so that you can stick to that five-minute time frame? If we need to change the time it takes to make a meal, can we do anything in advance to speed up the process – for example, cooking wholegrain rice in advance and freezing it? Consider the following:

1. How much time do I currently need to prepare each meal (including breakfast, lunch, evening meal and any snacks)? If you are not sure, consider making a time log.

2. What are the first changes you are going to make to the diet? I usually suggest beginning with one meal at a time, and starting with the meal that is the easiest to change. And then, once you have that in place, try changing the next meal.

3. Think about how you can do little things the evening before to help with meal preparation the next day. It could be something like peeling onions or cooking rice, soaking beans or nuts, or cooking beans. You can also buy kitchen equipment such as slow cookers that can be on all day and then have a hot stew or soup ready for when you return home.

4. Think about bulk cooking. This is a bit of a skill because it takes quite a lot of effort. Some parents do bulk cooking at the weekend.

5. Make the changes a habit. Once it becomes a habit, it will be a lot easier to maintain.

How to Build a Meal

One of the easy ways of thinking about a meal is to think of a plate. The ratio of vegetables, grains, protein and fruit may vary between children, but the key components remain the same: protein, carbohydrates and good-quality fat. Although varying rations may mean a child eats more vegetables or more protein or carbohydrates, the important thing to keep in mind is both the nutrient and energy content. Although there are not-one-rule-fits-all guidelines, here are some that can be used as a starting point.

Fruits and Vegetables

Fill half of the plate with fruits and vegetables. Fruits and vegetables should be washed well with water, lemon juice or a couple of drops of grapeseed extract. Although organic and fresh fruit and vegetables are best, frozen can be a time-saver.

Protein

A portion of protein for a child is the size of their hand. Protein may include meat, fish, eggs, beans or legumes, nuts or mushrooms. Where a child is not vegetarian, to bulk the nutritional content combine plant proteins or fibres with meat, fish or eggs. This can include adding vegetable fibre to meat patties or homemade burgers (as meat contains no fibre), and can be done without significantly affecting the texture of the meat product. For example, up to a fifth of pureéd sugar snap peas or kale pulp from juicing can be added, depending on your child's ability to tolerate them.

Starchy Carbohydrates

The US *MyPlate* suggests a little more than a quarter of grains or grain-like foods such as quinoa or buckwheat. These can be minimally processed, such as wholegrain basmati rice or sweet potato wedges. You can pack rice with plenty of vegetables; for example, mixing butternut squash with basmati rice or courgette (zucchini) noodles with rice noodles are ways to sneak in more vegetables and to increase nutritional density.

Fat

Any fat that is added to the meal should ideally be of the highest quality – virgin, organic and minimally processed. And where possible, you can do the processing yourself with high-fat foods such as seed milks or nut butters, or dips made from avocado, seeds or nuts. These include the natural protective antioxidants as well as the fibre necessary to increase nutritional density and to protect the food in the body.

Building Breakfast

Breakfast options should include a protein choice, a naturally high-fibre wholefood such as wholegrains, fruits or vegetables and a natural high-quality fat.

1. Choose protein such as egg, avocado, green beans, almonds, seeds, sausages or yoghurt.

2. Choose a naturally high-fibre wholegrain or grain-like food such as wholegrain rice, rolled oats, quinoa, millet, buckwheat, amaranth or teff. These come as wholegrains, as flakes and puffed. Cooking them from whole is a good choice. You can then mill them into porridge. This can be done in a slow cooker overnight, or by putting them on the stove to cook in the morning when you wake up, so that they are ready by breakfast time. You can also soak any of these grains or pseudo-grains overnight to make them easier to cook and digest when eaten. Puffed grains/pseudo-grains have the highest GI, so can be combined with a lower GI milk choice, seeds, nuts or coconut, depending on the child's needs.

3. Choose 1–3 portions of fruits or vegetables. Examples include one chopped fig, ten blueberries and ten raspberries, or the equivalent of your child's handfuls of raspberries and blueberries. You can choose low sugar fruits, such as limes, lemons, rhubarb, raspberries or blackberries.

4. Add a teaspoon of high-quality fat, such as a nut oil, seed oil, hemp oil, flax oil, extra virgin olive oil, virgin safflower or virgin coconut oil to your breakfast.

Table 9.1: Nutritional content of different fruits

Food name	Qty (g)	Measure	Starch	Fibre	Sugars	Glucose	Fructose	Sucrose	GI (est)
Dates (dried)	28.4	4	0	0	19.3	10.1	9.3	0	17.6
Bananas, weighed with skin	104	Small	1.6	2.1	14.4	3.3	3.4	7.6	54
Raisins	18	1 tbsp	0	1.1	12.5	6.2	6.3	0	115
Pears, raw, average	115	Small	0	3.2	11.5	2.6	8.2	0.8	44
Melon, honeydew	130	Average slice	0	1.2	8.6	3.6	4.2	0.8	85
Apples, eating, raw	67	Small	0	1.4	7.9	1.1	4.2	2.6	25
Grapes	50	Average portion	0	0.4	7.7	3.8	3.9	0.1	23
Cherries, raw	77	Average portion	0	0.9	7.3	3.8	3.4	0.2	16.9
Kiwi fruit	60	1 medium	0.2	1.4	6.2	2.8	2.6	0.8	32
Strawberries, raw	97	Average portion	0	1.9	5.8	2.5	2.9	0.3	24
Mangoes, ripe, raw	40	1 slice	0.1	1.2	5.5	0.3	1.2	4	20
Sweet potato	65	½ small	7.8	1.4	5.5	0	0	0	61
Peaches, raw	70	Small	0	1.6	5.3	0.8	0.8	3.6	29
Plums, raw	30	Small	0	0.7	2.6	1.3	0.6	0.8	11.7
Tomatoes, raw	85	Small	0	1.1	2.6	1.2	1.3	0.1	15
Carrots, raw	30	½ carrot	0.1	0.8	1.7	0.5	0.5	0.7	16
Courgette (zucchini), in blended oil	40	Small portion	0	0.8	1	0.4	0.5	0.1	15
Bilberries or blueberries	30	15	0	0.8	2.1	1	1	0.1	6
Blackberries, raw	30	6	0	2	1.5	0.8	0.8	0	6

Table 9.2: Examples of breakfast

Breakfast 1	Breakfast 2	Breakfast 3
1 tbsp Cashew Nut Cream	Sausages	Yoghurt
Porridge oats	Sweet potato	Puffed amaranth
Blueberries	Avocado	Plum
1 tsp coconut oil	Extra virgin olive oil	Sunflower seeds

Building Lunch or an Evening Meal

Lunch and evening meals follow a similar pattern. Options should include a protein choice, a naturally high-fibre wholefood such as wholegrains, fruit or vegetables and a natural high-quality fat. Some families may follow a grain-free diet to avoid starchy carbohydrates. In this case, it is worth remembering that starchy carbohydrates contain more energy than vegetables, so when you reduce starchy carbohydrates, energy and nutrients will have to come from another source. Chapters 5 and 6 give plenty of ideas for recipes that can be used as part of a supernourishing diet.

1. Choose protein, such as nuts, seeds, legumes (e.g. lentils), eggs, fish, meat or dairy (ricotta, mascarpone, goat's or sheep's cheese).

2. Choose a naturally high-fibre wholegrain or grain-like food such as wholegrain rice, rolled oats, quinoa, millet, buckwheat, amaranth or teff, wholewheat pasta and noodles, or potatoes in their skins (new potatoes rather than sweet potatoes).

3. Try to choose green vegetables where you can at every lunch and evening meal. Examples of green vegetables include kale, bok choy, watercress, lamb's lettuce or other lettuce, rocket and broccoli. If your child avoids green vegetables, try something white or colourful. Examples of white and colourful vegetables include cauliflower, turnip, parsnips, radish, celeriac, swede, carrots, pumpkin and butternut squash. Add foods from the onion family, such as onions, garlic, spring onions (scallions), leeks or chives.

4. Add a teaspoon of a high-quality fat, such as nut oil, seed oil, hemp oil, flax oil, extra virgin olive oil, virgin safflower oil or virgin coconut oil to your meal.

Table 9.3: Examples of lunch/evening meal

Lunch/evening meal 1	Lunch/evening meal 2	Lunch/evening meal 3
Lean mince (ground meat)	Rocket pesto	Pancake wrap sandwich
Kale	New potatoes	Hummus
Onion and garlic	Salmon	Avocado
Wholewheat spaghetti	Lettuce	Mustard cress
Extra virgin olive oil	Leeks	Grated carrots
		Spring onion (scallion)

Tips on Menu Planning

There are many ways to plan weekly or monthly menus. There are even apps and online menu-planning programmes. Or simply take a pencil and some paper. Choose what works for you. Below I give some tips on how to plan a menu, and things to consider.

1. Decide whether you will be making a plan for a week or a month. I would encourage you to plan for a week, and then learn what works and what doesn't work for you. Practise it a few times, tweaking it, and then use the successful parts of the plan to go on to plan for longer periods of time.

2. Alternatively, make a list like the one in Table 9.5. Add in any adjustments you are making to a given recipe. For example, if you are making fish pie and using celeriac mash instead of potatoes, write 'fish pie with celeriac mash'.

3. List the foods you choose under the meal-builder categories in Table 9.6 to ensure you have thought about all the components of a meal. For example, you could choose sausages (protein), sweet potato wedges (whole carbohydrate), green beans (green or colourful vegetable), garlic (onion family) and a homemade dip (high-quality fat).

4. Once you have brainstormed what meals you will be having in a week, list all the ingredients that each meal contains. Tick off all the foods that you already have in your cupboard or fridge. Use the remaining list as a shopping list.

5. Think also about when your child is away from home – do you need to buy any extras or prepare any foods so that your child does not feel left out?

6. Consider any pre-preparation you need to do, such as soaking rice or beans, or peeling and chopping. You can do this the evening before whilst you are watching television.

7. Finally, create a table containing the different meal/food choices for a given week, like the one shown in Table 9.7 below.

Table 9.4: Brainstorming meal ideas

Breakfast			
Cereal breakfasts	Pancakes, muffins or breads	Higher-protein-based breakfast	Fruit and nuts and yoghurt
Lunch/evening meal			
Meatless Monday or vegetarian	World cuisine (e.g. Mexican)	Soups or stir-fry or sandwich	Traditional dishes (e.g. shepherd's pie)
Snacks			
Muffins or crackers	Fruit or vegetable	Smoothie, juice	Ice pop or other

Table 9.5: Different types of meal, with adjustments

Breakfast	Lunch	Evening meal
Homemade sausage patties (made from mince (ground meat)) Yoghurt (see Cashew Nut Milk Yoghurt in Chapter 4) with grated carrots and chopped walnuts Butternut Squash and Papaya Millet Porridge with pumpkin seeds Millet granola with almond milk (add in 1 tsp coconut flour)	Lettuce fajitas Broccoli and pea soup and sweet potato Rice bowl (with salmon, brown rice and mayonnaise) Chicken sandwich with lettuce and cucumber	Fish pie (with celeriac mash) Pasta bake (gluten-free pasta) Spaghetti Bolognese (gluten-free pasta and extra vegetables – sweet potato) Bangers and mash (with swede and carrot mash) Shepherd's pie (with potato and celeriac mash)

Table 9.6: Different categories for food choices

Protein	Whole carbohydrate	Green or colourful vegetable	Onion family or fruit	High-quality fat

Table 9.7: Breakfast, lunch, evening meal and snacks for each day of the week

	Breakfast	Lunch	Evening meal	Snacks
Sunday				
Monday				
Tuesday				
Wednesday				
Thursday				
Friday				
Saturday				

There are many more options that you could choose, but keep it as simple as possible. Once you get used to menu planning, it will take far less time. It is worth the investment in planning a week's meal ahead, even if it means you just have it jotted down on a piece of paper.

Shopping for Food

Shopping can also be a bit of a chore. If you can't buy certain foods in the shops you normally visit, consider online shopping. This saves time and can make life a lot easier, not least because you do not need to keep creating a shopping list (after you have created your initial list). Online shopping also allows you to purchase more specialist food that may not be easily available elsewhere. It does cost extra to have groceries delivered, but then you don't have to spend money on travelling.

Buying Locally and in Season

Fresh and organic food bought locally through vegetable or fruit box schemes are a good idea. What I like about vegetable box schemes is that they use minimal plastic packaging from farm to kitchen. I have seen children improve simply by eating organic foods from such box schemes. Also, the food will have been picked more recently, so its nutrient value should be at its highest.

If you live in an area with a local farmers' market, you could buy local food from there. The quality of the eggs from small local farms, for example, will be much better than supermarket-bought eggs.

Reading Food Labels

The ingredients list is the most important thing to read on a food product. It lists the specific ingredients that the food product contains, listed in order of quantity. For example, on a packet of cornflakes the list may begin with *maize*, *sugar* and then *flavouring*. This means that in cornflakes, maize is the largest ingredient, followed by sugar.

Sometimes the ingredients list will also contain ingredients that you may not recognize, possibly because of the descriptive word used, or because it is listed as an E-number. An E-number is a code that represents a food additive. It is best to avoid them because some people can be sensitive to them. Table 9.8 lists a range of descriptive words for different forms of sugars or sweeteners. Some food products will list cane sugar as an ingredient, followed by maltodextrin or barley malt. So being aware of different forms of sugars in a food product is important, especially if you are cutting down on sugars in the diet.

Table 9.8: Different types of sugars

Barley malt	Diatase	Maltodextrin
Beet sugar	Ethyl maltol	Maltose
Brown sugar	Fructose	Malt syrup
Buttered syrup	Fruit juice	Maple syrup
Cane juice crystals	Fruit juice concentrate	Molasses
Cane sugar	Galactose	Muscovado sugar
Caramel	Glucose	Panocha
Corn syrup	Glucose solids	Raw sugar
Corn syrup solids	Golden sugar	Refiner's syrup
Confectioner's sugar	Golden syrup	Rice syrup
Carob syrup	Grape sugar	Sorbitol
Caster sugar	High fructose corn syrup	Sorghum syrup
Date sugar	Honey	Sucrose
Demerara sugar	Icing sugar	Sugar
Dextran	Invert sugar	Treacle
Dextrose	Lactose	Turbinado sugar
Diastatic malt		Yellow sugar

Major allergens are often listed on food labels. These include milk, eggs, fish, shellfish, tree nuts, peanuts, soybeans and wheat, and in the UK, cereals containing gluten, milk, celery, mustard, sesame, sulphur dioxide and lupin. The UK government requires emphasis of these major allergens on the ingredient label through the use of bold, underline or highlighting. If there is a possibility of any cross-contamination, the labelling should include, for example, 'May contain nuts or milk'. Allergens can be listed in parenthesis, for example: 'Enriched flour (wheat flour, malted barley, niacin, thiamin)'. Or they can be listed under 'Contains', for example 'Contains: wheat, milk, egg and soy'.

Foods can only be labelled as gluten-free if there is less than 20 parts gluten per million. Cereals such as oats, which sometimes cause reactions in sub-groups of people with coeliac disease, can also be labelled as gluten-free if they are uncontaminated and contain less than 20 parts gluten per million. When following a gluten-free diet, even hidden forms of gluten need to be avoided (see Table 9.9).

Table 9.9: Different hidden ingredients that might contain gluten

Bouillon/stock cubes	Farina	Seasonings
Bread crumbs	Gravies	Seitan
Brewer's yeast	Hydrolyzed wheat protein	Semolina
Bulgur wheat	Ice cream (might contain	Soups
Cereals containing wheat,	cookie dough)	Sausages (may contain
rye, barley, non-gluten-free	Kamut	wheat or rusks)
oats and ingredients such as	Malt vinegar	Triticale
barley malt	Malted milk	Vegetarian meat alternatives
Chips (can be coated with	Malt syrup	Wheat flour
wheat flour)	Malt flavouring	Wheat germ
Durum	Matzo meal	Wheat starch
Einkorn	Modified wheat starch	
Emmer	Oatmeal	
Energy bars	Rye and rye bread	

Kitchen Equipment

Although having the right equipment in the kitchen can make life easier, easy comes with practice. Some of the items recommended here are expensive to buy, but are real time-savers, while other items, although lower in cost, will do the same job.

Blenders, Hand Blenders and Food Processors

I think the simplest blending tool is a hand blender, especially if you are making dips, smoothies or blending fruits or vegetables to add to different foods. It is simple to detach the blending arm; this makes it quick and easy to wash. Some hand blender kits come with a chopping bowl and lid. This allows you to chop vegetables, herbs, nuts and seeds.

If you are making smoothies or soups, a traditional jug blender is easier to use. A glass or BPA-free plastic jug is preferable. Some suggest buying a blender with a higher wattage due to better performance. Customer reviews and consumer magazines can help you choose the best blender. In the UK Kenwood is a good brand. I would also recommend Vitamix – although it is expensive, it is easy to use, with a little practice. It can pulverize fibre to next to nothing for those who have issues with fibre digestion. You should always put wet ingredients in first, followed by dry ingredients, to allow the blade to move more freely – friction of the blade can heat the food.

Food processors can be a little more tricky. A food processor with a shredding blade can be quite useful for shredding things like cabbages for sauerkraut, for example. Food processors are better at chopping and homogenizing, so making things like sunflower butter is easier in a food processor, although it can be quite a long process.

Dehydrators

I am a big fan of dehydrators. Dehydrators such as the Excalibur, or those where air is drawn from the back and the heat is distributed evenly across the shelves, are preferable to those that distribute heat from the centre. Dehydrators are designed to remove moisture from food. Some have temperature-control dials that allow you to dehydrate at lower temperatures, such as 48°C/118°F, preserving enzymes or allowing things to evaporate more quickly at higher temperatures.

Excalibur dehydrators have trays with mesh screens that can be removed for cleaning. Various sheets can also be purchased to cover the mesh trays, which can be used for purées or foods that contain a lot of moisture.

Vegetable crisps, biscuits, energy bars, veggie bars, eggless macaroons and many more snack-like options can be made in the dehydrator.

Glass pots

I have come to think that glass and iron pots are possibly the best options, but these can be difficult to source at times, and can be quite expensive. Good-quality stainless steel is another option, although there is some concern that those with a nickel sensitivity could react to this option. Aluminium and copper pots should be avoided.

Juicers

The two main types of juicers are centrifugal and masticating. Centrifugal juicers usually juice more quickly, shredding fruit or vegetables at high speeds, whilst separating the juice from the pulp. More nutrients are thought to be lost in this process than with the masticating juicers, resulting in greater levels of oxidative stress. These juices should be drunk straightaway.

Masticating juicers grind the fruit or vegetables into a paste through a mesh screen. They can juice things like greens much more easily, as well as softer fruits such as pineapple. The juice from these juicers is less subject to oxidative stress and is thought to be more nutrient-dense.

Knives

A good chopping knife is essential. In fact, a good sharp knife is fundamental. You may need to invest a little more money, but it is worth the extra money spent, as a good knife is a real time-saver. When buying a knife, it is important to see how it feels in your hand when you grip it.

The best type of chef's knife is made from carbon steel, a very tough type of metal. Chef's knives are usually forged from a single piece of metal, from the tip of the knife through to the handle. The typical length of a chef's knife is between 20–30cm (8–12 inches).

The cutting edge needs to be kept sharp. A sharp knife is safer than a blunt knife, as it cuts the food more easily, so that you do not need to use any extra effort. This can be done by buying a knife sharpener, honing a knife with a steel, or sending it off to be sharpened.

Mandolin

A mandolin can be good to slice or julienne vegetables. If you are making salads, stir-fries or fermented vegetables, it can be a real time-saver. It is simple to use and easy to clean, but not essential.

Mason Jars

These can be used for storing soups, juices and smoothies. They are also the type of jars in which you can make sauerkraut.

Nut-Milk Bag

Nut-milk bags are ideal for straining, juicing or sprouting. Alternatively, it could be cheaper to purchase a yard of muslin and to use it with a sieve to process nut milk.

Spiralizer

A spiralizer allows you to turn vegetables into noodle threads of different sizes. You can then use these as you would noodles or spaghetti.

Offset Spatula

An offset spatula can be used to flip pancakes or lift baked goods off baking trays. It is a little more versatile than a normal spatula.

Vegetable Peeler

Get a good vegetable peeler – it will save you hours.

Knife Skills

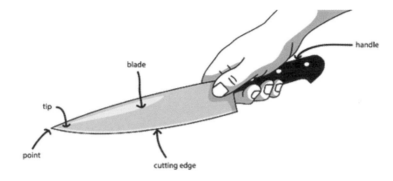

The Guiding Hand

When holding a chef's knife, there are a number of methods used. The image above shows the hand holding the knife. With the thumb on the blade, this improves the stability of the knife. The image on the right shows the hand that is not holding the knife. This is known as the guiding hand, and it holds the food steady. You need the food to 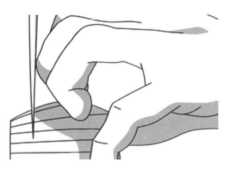 be steady when you are chopping and slicing for improved safety. You can see that the knuckle of the middle finger rests on the blade of the knife. The knuckle stabilizes the knife, helping to keep it upright.

Roll Slicing

Roll slicing is a technique used to slice up smaller vegetables and herbs. The types of vegetables that you could slice in this way include carrots, courgettes (zucchini) and small onions.

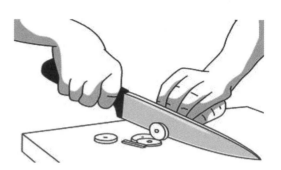

1. Hold the ingredients in a claw-like grip.

2. Holding the knife in your other hand, rest the knife against your knuckles. Place the tip on the board; lifting the heel of knife, push the knife down, tip to heel, in a rocking motion.

3. As you continue to slice the vegetable, adjust your guiding hand back on the food along the length of the ingredient. Continue slicing, keeping the tip of the knife on the board.

4. Keep the slices equal, and continue the rocking motion at a regular speed. Do not rush it; take your time. The more you practise, the more skilled you will become.

Chiffonade

Chiffonade uses the same slicing technique as roll slicing. The major difference is that you stack the vegetables (usually leaves) on top of each other, and then roll them up into a cigar-like shape. Examples of vegetables or herbs that you can chiffonade include lettuce, cabbage, kale, basil and spring onion (scallion).

1. Stack up the leaves, and roll into a cigar shape.

2. Follow the roll-slicing technique of a tip-to-heel rocking motion, to create equal slices.

Cross Chopping

This is used for ingredients that tend to have a more intense smell or flavour, such as herbs, onions and garlic. The aim is to chop the ingredients into small pieces of a similar size.

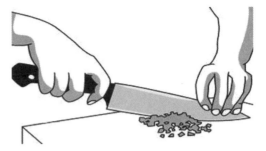

1. Hold the handle of the knife firmly.

2. Use your guiding hand on the top of the blade to stabilize the front end of the knife.

3. Hold the knife in this position and rock the heel and tip of the knife, keeping the tip of the knife in the same position, whilst rotating the back of the knife across the board.

Cutting

Ingredients can also be cut into longer slices or batons, and then chopped into dice or squares. These cuts need to be cut into equal lengths and widths to allow for uniform cooking. Carrots are commonly used to practise these cuts.

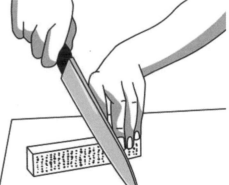

1. Peel the vegetable.

2. Slice off the edges of each side of the vegetable lengthways. (You can keep the edges to make soup.) This results in a long rectangular-shaped vegetable that does not roll around on the board.

3. The vegetable is now ready to slice into batons, julienne or other shapes.

Julienne

There are many different cuts of vegetables that are stick-shaped. One of the most common is julienne. This comes in two sizes – fine julienne and matchstick. Matchstick is 3mm × 3mm × 5cm (0.12 × 0.12 × 1.97 inches). Fine Julienne is 1.5cm × 1.5cm × 5cm (0.6 × 0.6 × 1.97 inches).

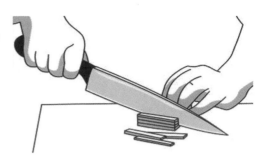

1. Once you have cut the vegetable into a baton, cut the baton to 5cm (1.97 inches) in length. Then cut through the vegetable, into 1.5cm (0.6 inch) slices.

2. Stack up the vegetables and cut into 1.5cm (0.6 inch) batons again.

Dicing

Dicing is when you cut the batons into cubes. These very fine cuts of vegetables can be used in different ways in the cooking process.

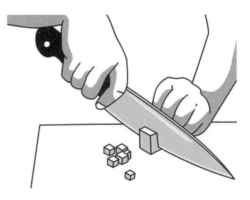

Petit brunoise is made from julienne – you line up the julienne, and chop the matchsticks into 3mm (0.12 inch) lengths so they can be cut into 3mm cubes. This technique can be used to make Mexican salsa, or for making a base, using carrots, onions and celery, for French and Italian soups.

Planning mealtimes, thinking about key meal-building foods, choosing recipes, and having the right ingredients in the house, all help to ensure that you are serving healthier foods, and make it more likely that you will stick to the plan. Having the right kitchen equipment also helps to speed the process. And if you like the process of cooking itself, getting a good knife will make vegetable preparation a pleasure. Remember when you are starting out that you may be out of your comfort zone, but practise, practise, practise until meal planning becomes second nature.

10 Strategies to Overcome Feeding Challenges and Changing Eating Habits

Leo liked to run around the room at mealtimes. It was a struggle to get him to eat. The food had to be placed on the plate in a particular way – different foods could not touch each other. Nothing green could be on the plate. So no broccoli, green beans, kale or peas. Leo's diet was restricted to mostly carbohydrate-rich foods like bread, pasta and rice cakes. And he only ate specific brands of fish fingers and chicken nuggets. Leo's case is all too common.

Running around at mealtimes is sometimes described as disruptive behaviour, and this was one of the three major feeding difficulties observed by William Ahearn, Director of Research from the New England Center for Children in the US.[108]

Feeding is a sensory-rich task. At mealtimes the colour and smell of the food on the plate sends a whirl of sensory information to the brain. Texture and taste then continue to stimulate the senses. The brain then needs to coordinate and integrate this information. Sometimes this makes the child feel overwhelmed, and there is the added challenge for a child of having to sit still whilst they eat. Knowing that children may have challenges with organizing and processing sensory information can help us to understand why they may need to run around during mealtimes. Understanding that the texture or smell of certain foods can be a challenge may help us to see why a child rejects certain foods.

Stephen is an adult with high-functioning autism. He explains that he did not eat tomatoes for a year following a negative eating experience. Tactile defensiveness, as it is called, is one of the potential drivers of selective eating and refusal of certain foods. According to Stephen: 'The sensory stimulation of having that small piece of fruit explode in my mouth was too much to bear, and I was not going to take any chances of it happening again.'[109]

Such texture sensitivity is thought to be present in up to 70 per cent of children with autism.

Another feeding challenge is problems with chewing and swallowing. Swallowing requires one of the most complicated, coordinated actions of muscle movement anywhere in the human body, involving 25 pairs of muscles in the mouth.[110] And this requires sufficient energy supply for it to work well.[111]

Pain or irritation in the throat can affect swallowing. Gastroesophageal reflux disease (GERD) is commonly reported in children with autism. GERD or acid reflux disease can be described as damage to the mucus layer in the oesophagus (the tube between the throat and stomach) as a result of stomach acid travelling back up the tube. This can cause irritation and pain, making eating a challenge. An infection such as strep throat is another possible factor influencing swallowing.[112]

Poor feeding patterns are related to feeding skills such as stuffing too much food into the mouth, thus increasing the chances of gagging, choking or drooling.

Insufficient food intake is a another major feeding difficulty – causes include refusing food, selective eating or eating a small range of foods or choosing from a narrow selection of food groups. Researchers comparing the eating behaviours of children with and without autism showed that those with autism were significantly more likely to have eating problems and that they ate a narrower range of foods than their neurotypical peers.[113] William et al.[114] evaluated 100 children with autism between the ages of 22 months and 10 years, and found that 67 per cent of these children were described as 'picky' eaters. Insufficient food intake or restricted food selection can influence overall energy and nutrient intake, and as a result, can affect physical development and cognitive function. It can also lead to borderline severe nutrient deficiencies, with extreme cases of nutrient deficiencies reported. A five-year-old boy only eating bacon, blueberry muffins and Kool-Aid® developed a bilateral corneal ulcer (an open sore in the outer layer of the cornea, the transparent layer on the front of the eye) due to vitamin A deficiency. We also observed patterns of nutritional deficiencies in the clinic.

So there are a number of reasons why children refuse or limit food intake. It is important to consider some of the possible triggers and symptoms associated with these triggers if they appear in your child. Understanding why your children eat in the way they do is also important. This is because malnutrition can occur, even if your child is a healthy weight.

All of the possible triggers and symptoms listed in Table 10.1 are to raise awareness of some of the challenges that children with autism can face that can affect their feeding. The list is not exhaustive but serves to give you some examples from which you can make further explorations. Some of these suggestions can be found in *Food Chaining: The Proven 6-Step Plan to Stop Picky Eating, Solve Feeding Problems and Expand Your Child's Diet.*[115] If your child is experiencing any of the symptoms on the list, or if you have concerns about any of the conditions listed, you should consult with relevant health professionals, such as your GP or physician.

Occupational and speech therapists, as well as physicians or GPs, are part of the multidisciplinary team needed to support children with these complex needs. Any complication due to poor feeding habits can lead to low weight, failure to thrive and other symptoms such as fatigue, irritability and light-headedness.

Sensory issues can also affect eating behaviour at the table, influencing behaviours such as running in circles rather than sitting at the table, poor hand-to-mouth coordination, or the child may be overwhelmed due to a colourful tablecloth. With all these sensory challenges, you should consider if there are any underlying issues.

Table 10.1: Possible triggers for symptoms associated with challenging eating habits in children

Possible triggers	Symptoms
Reflux Gastroesophageal reflux disease (GERD)	Vomiting Colic-like symptoms Spitting up Sore throat Choking or gagging Heartburn Regurgitation
Idiopathic eosinophilic oesophagitis (this is a condition where for an unknown reason there is an increase in white blood cells, known as eosinophils, in the tube between the mouth and the throat, known as the oesophagus)	Coughing Gagging Choking Vomiting Poor weight gain Eczema Hives Asthma
Constipation	Low appetite and passing stools fewer than three times a week
Strep throat	Refusing food Only eating soft or crunchy foods
An infection (e.g. a viral infection can promote oesophagitis)	Refusing food
Yeast overgrowth	Craving for particular sugary foods
Food sensitivities and intolerances	Rash or hives Lip swelling Runny nose, nasal congestion Eczema Abdominal pain Diarrhoea Vomiting Bloating Headaches
Taste sensitivities	Avoiding green leafy vegetables
Breathing difficulties Inflammation of the tonsils, such as tonsillitis	Problems swallowing
Weak oral motor muscles	Coughing Loud gulping as swallows Fatigue as eating progresses Need to swallow lots of times for a small amount of food Food left in mouth between teeth and inner cheek May not like eating textured foods such as meat Does not chew properly Chews food at front of mouth

Having addressed any medical concerns, we can consider some ideas to support picky eating (see Table 10.2).

Table 10.2: Different sensory issues at mealtimes

Sensory	Sensory experience	Tips
Auditory	Sounds reverberating from cafeteria walls at lunchtime. Children chattering, talking and screaming in the dinner hall.	Turn off electronics that give off sound such as televisions, computers and iPads at mealtimes. Eat in a quiet classroom.
Visual	Dislikes colour, prefers bland-coloured foods. Refuses foods if certain colours are on the plate.	Use calming colours such as green. Eat in naturally lit rooms or classrooms.
Taste and smell	Refuses spicy foods. Refuses strong-tasting foods. Gags at strong smells. Refuses to enter a room with a strong smell.	Choose bland-tasting foods (mashed potatoes are quite bland; if you wanted to add in another vegetable, only mix in a tiny amount at a time).
Touch	May try to remove food from plate. Gags when trying a new food.	May not like the texture of certain foods. May need to begin with textures that the child likes, and then increase the variety of foods.

One of the key things to consider with feeding problems is that you want mealtimes to have as low stress levels as possible. Many families feel that mealtimes can be quite challenging and frustrating, sometimes lasting over an hour if children refuse to eat. It can be especially frustrating when you have prepared a complex meal, and then the child refuses to eat it. Start with achievable goals to build the child's confidence, and also to manage your own frustration levels. It is best to work with an experienced feeding therapist to guide you at first. Remember that routine is key – try to make things as predictable as possible. Do not give up! Keep trying new foods.

Food Chaining and Other Methods

There are additional techniques that can be used to help children to include new foods in their diet. Food chaining is one example. It is 'based on the idea that your child will eat what he likes…a food chain introduces more foods that have similar flavours or features.'[116] If your child likes breaded foods, use the chain of chicken nuggets → fish fingers → breaded vegetables; if your child likes mayonnaise, use chicken nugget with mayonnaise → grilled chicken with mayonnaise → grilled fish with mayonnaise.

There are a number of techniques that underlie this method. These include flavour mapping, where you look at the flavours of the foods that your child enjoys. For example, if they like salty, sweet or spicy foods, look for foods that map that flavour. So if they like salty popcorn, for example, you could try salty parsnip crisps or salty celeriac chips. If they like sweet custard, you could try the Butternut Squash and Papaya Millett Porridge recipe from Chapter 5 and add extra honey. In terms of choosing more nourishing choices, you could flavour map, for example, providing food with equal sweetness at the beginning, and then gradually reducing the sweetness.

Flavour masking is using a condiment or sauce to mask a taste, such as tomato ketchup with broccoli.

Transitional foods are foods that are used to encourage a child to try a new food. These would include foods such as a bite of a potato crisp followed by a bite of a vegetable crisp. If you want to make the foods more nourishing, gradually increase the more nourishing food whilst reducing the less nourishing food.

Surprise foods are foods that are quite different from your child's usual food, where ideally you and your child put a dish together so your child can get used to the food and assemble the dish, for example, breaking up some nuts to add to yoghurt, or making a simple snack, like Cauliflower Popcorn (see Chapter 7).

Additional techniques include differential reinforcement, when a behaviour is rewarded immediately after it is done, so the child associates something positive with a specific behaviour. For example, if a child takes a bit of cauliflower mash, they get their iPad for two minutes.

Systematic desensitization is when you change the shape, colour, taste or texture of food. For example, for texture you might have raw carrot sticks, boiled carrots or carrot soup.

Becoming familiar with different methods, either through training, reading or working with an experienced feeding therapist, are all ways that can help to build the skills you need to support your child towards healthier and happier eating experiences.

To conclude, eating is a multi-sensory and complex task. It involves social, psychological and visual processing, as well as smell, taste, texture, sound and balance, and a lot of other sensory and psychological input. Children with autism can present with picky eating and nutritional deficiencies. As we simplify the diet and help to address any underlying issues, such as, for example, bacterial or yeast overgrowth, we would hope that some of these sensory issues would improve. But we must start at the baseline in attempting to understand what could be driving the behaviour we see at the dinner table, rather than assuming it is purely behavioural; and it is important to raise awareness of what types of things can trigger feeding difficulties.

Once we have evaluated the child for any health conditions, or weak oral motor muscles, we are in a better position to support the feeding process.

There are many forms of feeding therapy, and we recommend the help of skilled professionals.

This is, however, a much neglected area for children with autism and for children without autism with feeding difficulties. At the beginning of this chapter we saw some examples of severely restricted diets. In clinic I have seen a transformation from this type of diet to a diet rich in varied foods including vegetables – a supernourishing variety of foods that testify to the effectiveness of addressing the health issues behind the feeding difficulties combined with feeding therapy.

We encourage families of children with autism to persevere. Different individual families will be able to commit to varying levels of dietary change, but whatever you choose to commit to, remember that simple logic tells us that healthier foods and better digestion are likely to mean a healthier body. And if, as we continue to find out, the body and mind are linked, we hope this will also lead to a healthier body and a better functioning mind.

The final thing about habit change is that you don't need to try to change everything at once. You can start with one thing. Get into the habit of doing that one thing, and then add another change. Do not underestimate the power of little changes, because it is on the back of little changes working together that you get big change.

'The mind that opens to a new idea never returns to its original size.' (Albert Einstein)

NOTES

1. Bergström-Isacsson, M. (2011) 'Music and Vibroacoustic Stimulation in People with Rett Syndrome – A Neurophysiological Study.' PhD Thesis. Aalborg University, Denmark.
2. Gottschall, E. (1994) *Breaking the Vicious Cycle: Intestinal Health through Diet.* Baltimore, ON: The Kirkton Press.
3. Huston, J. (2012) 'The vagus nerve and the inflammatory reflex: wandering on a new treatment paradigm for systemic inflammation and sepsis.' *Surgical Infections 13*(4), 187–193. Metz, C. and Tracey, K. (2005) 'It takes nerve to dampen inflammation.' *Nature Immunology 6*(8), 756–758.
4. Gómez-Pinilla, F. (2008) 'Brain foods: the effects of nutrients on brain function.' *Nature Reviews Neuroscience 9*(7), 568–578. Strader, A. and Woods, S. (2005) 'Gastrointestinal hormones and food intake.' *Gastroenterology 128*(1), 175–191.
5. Collins, S., Surette, M. and Bercik, P. (2012) 'The interplay between the intestinal microbiota and the brain.' *Nature Reviews Microbiology 10*(11), 735–742. Cryan, J. and O'Mahony, S. (2011) 'The microbiome-gut–brain axis: from bowel to behavior.' *Neurogastroenterology & Motility 23*(3), 187–192.
6. Williams, B., Hornig, M., Buie, T., Bauman, M. *et al.* (2011) 'Impaired carbohydrate digestion and transport and mucosal dysbiosis in the intestines of children with autism and gastrointestinal disturbances.' *PloS One 6*(9), e24585.
7. Kanner, L. (1943) 'Autistic disturbances of affective contact.' *Nervous Child 2*(3), 217–250.
8. Levisohn, P. (2007) 'The autism–epilepsy connection.' *Epilepsia 48*(s9), 33–35.
9. APA (American Psychiatric Association) (1952) *Diagnostic and Statistical Manual of Mental Disorders.* Arlington, VA: APA.
10. Evans, B. (2013) 'How autism became autism: the radical transformation of a central concept of child development in Britain.' *History of the Human Sciences*, 8 May.
11. Daly, E., Ecker, C., Hallahan, B., Deeley, Q. *et al.* (2014) 'Response inhibition and serotonin in autism: a functional MRI study using acute tryptophan depletion.' *Brain 137*(9), 2600–2610. Whitaker-Azmitia, P. (1999) 'The discovery of serotonin and its role in neuroscience.' *Neuropsychopharmacology 21*, 2S–8S.
12. APA (American Psychiatric Association) (1994) *Diagnostic and Statistical Manual of Mental Disorders, Fourth Edition.* Arlington, VA: APA.
13. Kendell, R.E. (2001) 'The distinction between mental and physical illness.' *The British Journal of Psychiatry 178*, 490–493, p.491.
14. Thagard, P. (2000) *How Scientists Explain Disease.* Princeton, NJ: Princeton University Press.
15. Ringen, P., Engh, J., Birkenaes, A., Dieset, I. and Andreassen, O. (2014) 'Increased mortality in schizophrenia due to cardiovascular disease – a non-systematic review of epidemiology, possible causes, and interventions.' *Schizophrenia 5*, 137.
16. Dickerson, F., Kirkpatrick, B., Boronow, J., Stallings, C., Origoni, A. and Yolken, R. (2006) 'Deficit schizophrenia: association with serum antibodies to cytomegalovirus.' *Schizophrenia Bulletin 32*(2), 396–400. Yolken, R. and Torrey, E. (1995) 'Viruses, schizophrenia, and bipolar disorder.' *Clinical Microbiology Reviews 8*(1), 131–145.
17. Genuis, S.J. and Lobo, R.A. (2014) 'Gluten sensitivity presenting as a neuropsychiatric disorder.' *Gastroenterology Research and Practice* doi:10.1155/2014/293206. Jackson, J., Eaton, W., Cascella, N., Fasano, A. and Kelly, D. (2012) 'Neurologic and psychiatric manifestations of celiac disease and gluten sensitivity.' *Psychiatric Quarterly 83*(1), 91–102. Pynnönen, P., Isometsä, E., Verkasalo, M., Kähkönen, S. *et al.* (2005) 'Gluten-free diet may alleviate depressive and behavioural symptoms in adolescents with coeliac disease: a prospective follow-up case-series study.' *BMC Psychiatry 5*(1), 14.
18. Ghaziuddin, M., Tsai, L.Y., Eilers, L. and Ghaziuddin, N. (1992) 'Brief report: autism and herpes simplex encephalitis.' *Journal of Autism and Developmental Disorders 22*(1), 107–113. Gillberg, C. (1986) 'Brief report: onset at age 14 of a typical autistic syndrome. A case report of a girl with herpes simplex encephalitis.' *Journal of Autism and Developmental Disorders 16*(3), 369–375.

19. Gillberg, C. (1991) 'Autistic syndrome with onset at age 31 years: herpes encephalitis as a possible model for childhood autism.' *Developmental Medicine & Child Neurology 33*(10), 920–924.

20. Napoli, E., Dueñas, N. and Giulivi, C. (2014) 'Potential therapeutic use of the ketogenic diet in autism spectrum disorders.' *Frontiers in Pediatrics 2.* Whiteley, P., Haracopos, D., Knivsberg, A.-M., Reichelt, K. *et al.* (2010) 'The ScanBrit randomised, controlled, single-blind study of a gluten-and casein-free dietary intervention for children with autism spectrum disorders.' *Nutritional Neuroscience 13*(2), 87–100.

21. Millward, C., Ferriter, M., Calver, S. and Connell-Jones, G. (2008) 'Gluten- and casein-free diets for autistic spectrum disorder.' *Cochrane Database of Systematic Reviews 16*(2), April.

22. Ibid.

23. Panksepp, J. (1979) 'A neurochemical theory of autism.' *Trends in Neurosciences 2*, 174–177.

24. Puertollano, M., Puertollano, E., Alvarez de Cienfuegos, G. and de Pablo, M.A. (2011) 'Dietary antioxidants: immunity and host defense.' *Current Topics in Medicinal Chemistry 11*(14), 1752–1766.

25. Jackson, J., Eaton, W., Cascella, N., Fasano, A. and Kelly, D. (2012) 'Neurologic and psychiatric manifestations of celiac disease and gluten sensitivity.' *Psychiatric Quarterly 83*(1), 91–102.

26. Koletzko, S., Niggemann, B., Arato, A., Dias, J. *et al.* (2012) 'Diagnostic approach and management of cow's-milk protein allergy in infants and children: ESPGHAN GI Committee practical guidelines.' *Journal of Pediatric Gastroenterology and Nutrition 55*, 221–229.

27. Shepherd, S. and Gibson, P. (2011) *Food Intolerance: Management Plan.* Melbourne, VIC: Penguin Group. Williams, B., Hornig, M., Buie, T., Bauman, M. *et al.* (2011) 'Impaired carbohydrate digestion and transport and mucosal dysbiosis in the intestines of children with autism and gastrointestinal disturbances.' *PloS One 6*(9), e24585.

28. de Magistris, L., Familiari, V., Pascotto, A., Sapone, A. P. *et al.* (2010) 'Alterations of the intestinal barrier in patients with autism spectrum disorders and in their first-degree relatives.' *Journal of Pediatric Gastroenterology and Nutrition 51*(4), 418–424.

29. Casanova, M. (2007) 'The neuropathology of autism.' *Brain Pathology 17*(4), 422–433. Skefos, J., Cummings, C., Enzer, K., Holiday, J. *et al.* (2014) 'Regional alterations in Purkinje cell density in patients with autism.' *PloS One 9*(2), e81255. Vojdani, A., O'Bryan, T., Green, J., McCandless, J. *et al.* (2004) 'Immune response to dietary proteins, gliadin and cerebellar peptides in children with autism.' *Nutritional Neuroscience 7*(3), 151–161.

30. Mulloy, A., Lang, R., O'Reilly, M., Sigafoos, J., Lancioni, G. and Rispoli, M. (2010) 'Gluten-free and casein-free diets in the treatment of autism spectrum disorders: a systematic review.' *Research in Autism Spectrum Disorders 4*(3), 328–339. White, J. (2003) 'Intestinal pathophysiology in autism.' *Experimental Biology and Medicine 228*(6), 639–649.

31. Mass, M., Kubera, M. and Leunis, J. (2008) 'The gut–brain barrier in major depression: intestinal mucosal dysfunction with an increased translocation of LPS from gram negative enterobacteria (leaky gut) plays a role in the inflammatory pathophysiology of depression.' *Neuroendocrinology Letters 29*(1), 117–124. Theoharides, T., Asimenia, A., Konstantinos-Dionysios, A., Bodi, Z. *et al.* (2012) 'Mast cell activation and autism.' *Biochimica et Biophysica Acta (BBA)-Molecular Basis of Disease 1822*(1), 34-41.

32. Shah, J., Trivedi, M., Hodgson, N. and Deth, R. (2013) 'Casein and gluten-derived opiate peptides affect cysteine uptake and redox status.' *The FASEB Journal 27*, 1075.1.

33. Belobrajdic, D. and Bird, A. (2013) 'The potential role of phytochemicals in wholegrain cereals for the prevention of type-2 diabetes.' *Nutrition Journal 12*, 62. Liu, R.H. (2007) 'Whole grain phytochemicals and health.' *Journal of Cereal Science 46*(3), 207–219.

34. Lattimer, J. and Haub, M. (2010) 'Effects of dietary fiber and its components on metabolic health.' *Nutrients 2*(12), 1266–1289.

35. Al-Gadani, Y., El-Ansary, A., Attas, O. and Al-Ayadhi, L. (2009) 'Metabolic biomarkers related to oxidative stress and antioxidant status in Saudi autistic children.' *Clinical Biochemistry 42*(10), 1032–1040. Chauhan, A., Chauhan, V., Brown, W. and Cohen, I. (2004) 'Oxidative stress in autism: increased lipid peroxidation and reduced serum levels of ceruloplasmin and transferrin – the antioxidant proteins.' *Life Sciences 75*(21), 2539–2549.

36. Valacchi, G., Pecorelli, A., Signorini, C., Leoncini, S. *et al.* (2014) '4HNE Protein Adducts in Autistic Spectrum Disorders: Rett Syndrome and Autism.' In V.B. Patel, V.R. Preedy and C.R. Martin (eds) *Comprehensive Guide to Autism* (pp.2667–2687). New York: Springer.

37. Rose, S., Melnyk, S., Pavliv, O., Bai, S. *et al.* (2012) 'Evidence of oxidative damage and inflammation associated with low glutathione redox status in the autism brain.' *Translational Psychiatry 2*(7), e134. Welsh J., Ahn, E. and Placantonakis, D. (2005) 'Is autism due to brain desynchronization?' *International Journal of Developmental Neuroscience 23*(2), 253–263.

38. Emond, A., Emmett, P., Steer, C. and Golding, J. (2010) 'Feeding symptoms, dietary patterns, and growth in young children with autism spectrum disorders.' *Pediatrics 126*(2), e337–e342.

39. Higdon, J., Delage, B., Williams, D. and Dashwood, R. (2007) 'Cruciferous vegetables and human cancer risk: epidemiologic evidence and mechanistic basis.' *Pharmacological Research 55*(3), 224–236. Michaud, D., Pietinen, P., Taylor, P., Virtanen, M., Virtamo, J. and Albanes, D. (2002) 'Intakes of fruits and vegetables, carotenoids and vitamins A, E, C in relation to the risk of bladder cancer in the ATBC cohort study.' *British Journal of Cancer 87*(9), 960–965.

40. Mein, J., James, D. and Lakkanna, S. (2012) 'Induction of phase 2 antioxidant enzymes by broccoli sulforaphane: perspectives in maintaining the antioxidant activity of vitamins A, C, and E.' *Nutrigenomics 3*, 7.

41. Divyakolu, S., Tejaswini, Y., Thomas, W., Thumoju *et al.* (2013) 'Evaluation of C677T polymorphism of the methylenetetrahydrofolate reductase (MTHFR) gene in various neurological disorders.' *Journal of Neurological Disorders 2*(142).

42. Caudill, M.A. (2010) 'Folate bioavailability: implications for establishing dietary recommendations and optimizing status.' *The American Journal of Clinical Nutrition 91*(5), 1455S–1460S.

43. Schreck, K.A. and Williams, K. (2006) 'Food preferences and factors influencing food selectivity for children with autism spectrum disorders.' *Research in Developmental Disabilities 27*(4), 353–363.

44. Gómez-Pinilla, F. (2008) 'Brain foods: the effects of nutrients on brain function.' *Nature Reviews Neuroscience 9*(7), 568–578. McGinnis, W., Audhya, T. and Edelson, S. (2013) 'Proposed toxic and hypoxic impairment of a brainstem locus in autism.' *International Journal of Environmental Research and Public Health 10*(12), 6955–7000.

45. Mozaffarian, D., Pischon, T., Hankinson, S.E., Rifai, N. *et al.* (2004) 'Dietary intake of trans fatty acids and systemic inflammation in women.' *The American Journal of Clinical Nutrition 79*(4), 606–612.

46. Jaarin, K., Mustafa, M. and Leong, X. (2011) 'The effects of heated vegetable oils on blood pressure in rats.' *Clinics 66*(12), 2125–2132.

47. Dhaka, V., Gulia, N., Ahlawat, K. and Khatkar, B. (2011) 'Trans fats – sources, health risks and alternative approach – a review.' *Journal of Food Science and Technology 48*(5), 534–541.

48. Hediger, M., England, L., Molloy, C., Kai, F., Manning-Courtney, P. and Mills, J. (2008) 'Reduced bone cortical thickness in boys with autism or autism spectrum disorder.' *Journal of Autism and Developmental Disorders 38*(5), 848–856.

49. Ibid.

50. Kneen, R. and Solomon, T. (2008) 'Management and outcome of viral encephalitis in children.' *Paediatrics and Child Health 18*(1), 7–16.

51. Ames, B., Atamna, H. and Killilea, D. (2005) 'Mineral and vitamin deficiencies can accelerate the mitochondrial decay of aging.' *Molecular Aspects of Medicine 26*(4), 363–378. Ashoori, M. and Saedisomeolia, A. (2014) 'Riboflavin (vitamin B) and oxidative stress: a review.' *British Journal of Nutrition 111*(11), 1985–1991. Bates, C. (2005) 'Riboflavin.' In L. Allen, A. Prentice and A. Caballero (eds) *Encyclopedia of Human Nutrition* (four-volume set, 2nd edn). San Diego, CA: Academic Press. Fahmy, S., El-Hamamsy, M., Zaki, O. and Badary, O. (2013) 'l-carnitine supplementation improves the behavioral symptoms in autistic children.' *Research in Autism Spectrum Disorders 7*(1), 159–166. Hoey, L., McNulty, H. and Strain, J. (2009) 'Studies of biomarker responses to intervention with riboflavin: a systematic review.' *The American Journal of Clinical Nutrition*, ajcn-27230B. Madrigal, J., Olivenza, R., Moro, M., Lizasoain, I. *et al.* (2001) 'Glutathione depletion, lipid peroxidation and mitochondrial dysfunction are induced by chronic stress in rat brain.' *Neuropsychopharmacology 24*(4), 420–429. Meister, A. (1992) 'On the antioxidant effects of ascorbic acid and glutathione.' *Biochemical Pharmacology 44*(10), 1905–1915. Mythri, R., Jagatha, B., Pradhan, N., Andersen, J. and Bharath, M. (2007) 'Mitochondrial complex I inhibition in Parkinson's disease: how can curcumin protect mitochondria?' *Antioxidants & Redox Signaling 9*(3), 399–408. Pieczenik, S. and Neustadt, J. (2007) 'Mitochondrial dysfunction and molecular pathways of disease.' *Experimental and Molecular Pathology 83*(1), 84–92. Tang, Y., Gao, C., Xing, M., Li, Y. *et al.* (2012) 'Quercetin prevents ethanol-induced dyslipidemia and mitochondrial oxidative damage.' *Food and Chemical Toxicology 50*(5), 1194–1200. Tebib, K., Rouanet, J.M. and Besancon, P. (1997) 'Antioxidant effects of dietary polymeric grape seed tannins in tissues of rats fed a high cholesterol-vitamin E-deficient diet.' *Food Chemistry 59*(1), 135–141. Ungvari, Z., Sonntag, W., de Cabo, R., Baur, J. and Csiszar, A. (2011) 'Mitochondrial protection by resveratrol.' *Exercise and Sport Sciences Reviews 39*(3), 128. Wu, G., Fang, Y., Yang, S., Lupton, J. and Turner, N. (2004) 'Glutathione metabolism and its implications for health.' *The Journal of Nutrition 134*(3), 489–492.

52. Ulluwishewa, D., Anderson, R., McNabb, W., Moughan, P., Wells, J. and Roy, N. (2011) 'Regulation of tight junction permeability by intestinal bacteria and dietary components.' *The Journal of Nutrition 141*(5), 769–776.

53. Lam, K. and Chi-Keung Cheung, P. (2013) 'Non-digestible long chain beta-glucans as novel prebiotics.' *Bioactive Carbohydrates and Dietary Fibre 2*(1), 45–64. Vctvicka, V. (2014) 'Effects of β-glucan on some environmental toxins: an overview.' *Biomed Papers* 158(1), 1–4.

54. Rose, S., Melnyk, S., Pavliv, O., Bai, S. *et al.* (2012) 'Evidence of oxidative damage and inflammation associated with low glutathione redox status in the autism brain.' *Translational Psychiatry 2*(7), e134.

55. Mein, J., James, D. and Lakkanna, S. (2012) 'Induction of phase 2 antioxidant enzymes by broccoli sulforaphane: perspectives in maintaining the antioxidant activity of vitamins A, C, and E.' *Nutrigenomics 3*, 7. Yi, B., Kasai, H., Lee, H.-S., Kang, Y, Park, J. and Yang, M. (2011) 'Inhibition by wheat sprout (Triticum aestivum) juice of bisphenol A-induced oxidative stress in young women.' *Mutation Research/Genetic Toxicology and Environmental Mutagenesis 724*(64–68).

56. Liu, R.H. (2013) 'Health-promoting components of fruits and vegetables in the diet.' *Advances in Nutrition: An International Review Journal 4*(3), 384S–392S.

57. Shepherd, S. and Gibson, P. (2013) *The Complete Low-FODMAP Diet: A Revolutionary Plan for Managing IBS and Other Digestive Disorders.* New York: The Experiment LLC.

58. Duerkop, B.A., Vaishnava, S. and Hooper, L. (2009) 'Immune responses to the microbiota at the intestinal mucosal surface.' *Immunity 31*(3), 368–376.

59. Kwok, C., Arthur, A., Anibueze, C., Singh, S., Cavallazzi, R. and Loke, Y. (2012) 'Risk of Clostridium difficile infection with acid suppressing drugs and antibiotics: meta-analysis.' *The American Journal of Gastroenterology 107*(7), 1011–1019. Parracho, H., Bingham, M., Gibson, G. and McCartney, A. (2005) 'Differences between the gut microflora of children with autistic spectrum disorders and that of healthy children.' *Journal of Medical Microbiology 54*(10), 987–991.

60. Hartzell, S. and Seneff, S. (2012) 'Impaired sulfate metabolism and epigenetics: is there a link in autism?' *Entropy 14*(10), 1953–1977.

61. Barrett, J.S. and Gibson, P. (2012) 'Fermentable oligosaccharides, disaccharides, monosaccharides and polyols (FODMAPs) and nonallergic food intolerance: FODMAPs or food chemicals?' *Therapeutic Advances in Gastroenterology 5*(4), 261–268. Race, S. (2012) *The Salicylate Handbook: Your Guide to Understanding Salicylate Sensitivity.* Tigmor Books.

62. Neveu, V., Perez-Jiménez, J., Vos, F., Crespy, V. *et al.* (2010) 'Phenol-explorer: an online comprehensive database on polyphenol contents in foods.' *Database.* Rothwell, J., Urpi-Sarda, M., Boto-Ordoñez, M., Knox, C. *et al.* (2012) 'Phenol-Explorer 2.0: a major update of the Phenol-Explorer database integrating data on polyphenol metabolism and pharmacokinetics in humans and experimental animals.' *Database.* Rothwell, J., Pérez-Jiménez J., Neveu, V., Medina-Ramon, A. *et al.* (2013) 'Phenol-Explorer 3.0: a major update of the Phenol-Explorer database to incorporate data on the effects of food processing on polyphenol content.' *Database.*

63. Konstantynowicz, J., Porowski, T., Zoch-Zwierz, W., Wasilewska, J. *et al.* (2012) 'A potential pathogenic role of oxalate in autism.' *European Journal of Paediatric Neurology 16*(5), 485–491.

64. Ibid.

65. EFSA Panel on Biological Hazards (2011) 'Scientific opinion on risk based control of biogenic amine formation in fermented foods.' *EFSA Journal 9*(10), 2393.

66. von Bibra, H., Wulf, G., St John Sutton, M., Pfützner, A., Schuster, T. and Heilmeyer, P. (2014) 'Low-carbohydrate/high-protein diet improves diastolic cardiac function and the metabolic syndrome in overweight-obese patients with type 2 diabetes.' *IJC Metabolic & Endocrine 2*, 11–18.

67. Pennesi, C. and Klein, L.C. (2012) 'Effectiveness of the gluten-free, casein-free diet for children diagnosed with autism spectrum disorder: based on parental report.' *Nutritional Neuroscience 15*(2), 85–91.

68. Dodu, K. and Whiteley, P. (2014) 'Non-coeliac gluten sensitivity – a look at the evidence behind the headlines.' *Pharmaceutical Journal 292*, 292. Lau, N.M., Green, P.H., Taylor, A.K., Hellberg, D. *et al.* (2013) 'Markers of celiac disease and gluten sensitivity in children with autism.' *PloS One 8*(6), e66155.

69. Khwanchai, P., Chinprahast, N., Pichyangkura, R. and Chaiwanichsiri, S. (2014) 'Gamma-aminobutyric acid and glutamic acid contents, and the GAD activity in germinated brown rice (Oryza sativa L.): effect of rice cultivars.' *Food Science and Biotechnology 23*(2), 373–379.

70. Chai, W. and Liebman, M. (2005) 'Oxalate content of legumes, nuts and grain-based flours.' *Journal of Food Composition and Analysis 18*, 723–729.

71. Restani, P., Beretta, B., Fiocchi, A., Ballabio, C. and Galli, C. (2002) 'Cross-reactivity between mammalian proteins.' *Annals of Allergy, Asthma & Immunology 89*(6), 11–15.

72. Brostoff, J. and Gamlin, L. (1998) *Complete Guide to Food Allergy and Intolerance.* Leicester: Blitz.

73. Cheung, W., Zhan, J., Paik, K. and Mak, R. (2011) 'The impact of inflammation on bone mass in children.' *Pediatric Nephrology 26*(11), 1937–1946.

74. Daley, C.A., Abbott, A., Doyle, P.S., Nader, G.A. and Larson, S. (2010) 'A review of fatty acid profiles and antioxidant content in grass-fed and grain-fed beef.' *Nutrition Journal 9*(1), 10.

75. de la Monte, S., Tong, M. and Wands, J. (2011) 'Insulin resistance, cognitive impairment and neurodegeneration: roles of nitrosamine exposure, diet and lifestyles. Alzheimer's disease pathogenesis-core concepts, shifting paradigms and therapeutic targets.' *InTech, Rijeka, Croatia*, 459–496.

76. Fahey, J.W., Zhang, Y. and Talalay, P. (1997) 'Broccoli sprouts: an exceptionally rich source of inducers of enzymes that protect against chemical carcinogens.' *Proceedings of the National Academy of Sciences 94*(19), 10367–10372.

77. Yi, B., Kasai, H., Lee, H.-S., Kang, Y, Park, J. and Yang, M. (2011) 'Inhibition by wheat sprout (Triticum aestivum) juice of bisphenol A-induced oxidative stress in young women.' *Mutation Research/Genetic Toxicology and Environmental Mutagenesis 724* (64–68).

78. Micha, R., Michas, G. and Mozaffarian, D. (2012) 'Unprocessed red and processed meats and risk of coronary artery disease and type 2 diabetes – an updated review of the evidence.' *Current Atherosclerosis Reports 14*(6), 515–524.

79. Guran, H. and Oksuztepe, G. (2013) 'Detection and typing of Clostridium perfringens from retail chicken meat parts.' *Letters in Applied Microbiology 57*(1), 77–82.

80. Sabah, J., Juneja, V. and Fung, D. (2004) 'Effect of spices and organic acids on the growth of Clostridium perfringens during cooling of cooked ground beef.' *Journal of Food Protection 67*(9), 1840–1847.

81. US Food and Drug Administration (2014) 'Mercury levels in commercial fish and shellfish (1990–2010).' Available at www.fda.gov/food/foodborneillnesscontaminants/metals/ucm115644.htm, accessed on 1 June 2015.

82. Heath, A. (1995) *Water Pollution and Fish Physiology* (2nd edn). Boca Raton, FL: CRC Press.

83. US Food and Drug Administration (2014) 'Mercury levels in commercial fish and shellfish (1990–2010).' Available at www.fda.gov/food/foodborneillnesscontaminants/metals/ucm115644.htm, accessed on 1 June 2015.

84. Campos-Vega, R., Loarca-Piña, G. and Oomah, B. (2010) 'Minor components of pulses and their potential impact on human health.' *Food Research International 43*(2), 461–482.

85. Hartman, T., Albert, P., Zhang, Z., Bagshaw, D. *et al.* (2010) 'Consumption of a legume-enriched, low-glycemic index diet is associated with biomarkers of insulin resistance and inflammation among men at risk for colorectal cancer.' *The Journal of Nutrition 140*(1), 60–67.

86. Zhang, C., Monk, J., Lu, J., Zarepoor, L. *et al.* (2014) 'Cooked navy and black bean diets improve biomarkers of colon health and reduce inflammation during colitis.' *British Journal of Nutrition 111*(9), 1549–1563.

87. Neveu, V., Perez-Jiménez, J., Vos, F., Crespy, V. *et al.* (2010) 'Phenol-explorer: an online comprehensive database on polyphenol contents in foods.' *Database*. Rothwell, J., Urpi-Sarda, M., Boto-Ordoñez, M., Knox, C. *et al.* (2012) 'Phenol-Explorer 2.0: a major update of the Phenol-Explorer database integrating data on polyphenol metabolism and pharmacokinetics in humans and experimental animals.' *Database*. Rothwell, J., Pérez-Jiménez J., Neveu, V., Medina-Ramon, A. *et al.* (2013) 'Phenol-Explorer 3.0: a major update of the Phenol-Explorer database to incorporate data on the effects of food processing on polyphenol content.' *Database*.

88. Danczak, E. (2004) 'Glucosamine and plant lectins in autistic spectrum disorders: an initial report on six children with uncontrolled diarrhoea.' *Journal of Nutritional and Environmental Medicine 14*(4), 327–330. Sinha, N., Hui, Y., Evranuz, E., Siddiq, M. and Ahmed, J. (2010) *Handbook of Vegetables and Vegetable Processing*. Hoboken, NJ: Wiley-Blackwell. Siddiq, M., and Uebersax M. A. (eds) (2012) *Dry Beans and Pulses: Production, Processing and Nutrition*. London: John Wiley and Sons.

89. Chai, W. and Liebman, M. (2005) 'Oxalate content of legumes, nuts and grain-based flours.' *Journal of Food Composition and Analysis 18*, 723–729.

90. Katragadda, H.R., Fullana, A., Sidhu, S. and Carbonell-Barrachina, Á.A. (2010) 'Emissions of volatile aldehydes from heated cooking oils.' *Food Chemistry 120*(1), 59–65.

91. Rumsey, J.M., Duara, R., Grady, C. *et al.* (1985) 'Brain metabolism in autism: resting cerebral glucose utilization as measured with positron emission tomography (PET).' *Archives of General Psychiatry 42*, 448–455.

92. Patil, S. and Khan, M. (2011) 'Germinated brown rice as a value added rice product: a review.' *Journal of Food Science and Technology 48*(6), 661–667.

93. Twachtman-Reilly, J., Amaral, S. and Zebrowski, P. (2008) 'Addressing feeding disorders in children on the autism spectrum in school-based settings: physiological and behavioral issues.' *Language, Speech, and Hearing Services in Schools 39*(2), 261–272, p.262.

94. Canadian Cancer Society (2014) 'Cured, smoked and salt-preserved foods.' Available at www.cancer.ca/en/cancer-information/cancer-101/what-is-a-risk-factor/diet/cured-smoked-and-salt-preserved-foods/?region=on, accessed on 1 June 2015.

95. Kenney, M., Baird, M. and Winegard, S. (2014) *Plant Food*. Layton, UT: Gibbs Smith.

96. Annalisa, L., Costa, C., Conte, A. and Del Nobile, M.A. (2012) 'Food applications of natural antimicrobial compounds.' *Frontiers in Microbiology 3.* Sabah, J.R., Juncja, V.K. and Fung, D.Y.C. (2004) 'Effect of spices and organic acids on the growth of Clostridium perfringens during cooling of cooked ground beef.' *Journal of Food Protection 67*(9), 1840–1847. Harvey, R.B., Norman, K.N., Andrews, K., Norby, B. et al. (2011) 'Clostridium difficile in retail meat and processing plants in Texas.' *Journal of Veterinary Diagnostic Investigation 23*(4), 807–811.

97. Fuhrman, J. (2012) *Nutritarian Handbook and ANDI Food Scoring Guide.* Flemington, NJ: Gift of Health Press.

98. Garaulet, M. and Gómez-Abellán, P. (2014) 'Timing of food intake and obesity: a novel association.' *Physiology & Behavior 134*, 44–50.

99. Scott-Ricci, S. and Kyle, T. (2008) *Maternity and Pediatric Nursing.* Philadelphia, PA: Lippincott Williams & Wilkins.

100. Biesalski, H., Bischoff, S., Boehles, H., Muehlhoefer, A. and Working Group for Developing the Guidelines for Parenteral Nutrition of the German Association for Nutritional Medicine (2009) 'Water, Electrolytes, Vitamins and Trace Elements – Guidelines on Parenteral Nutrition.' *GMS German Medical Science 7*, Chapter 7. Popkin, B., D'Anci, K. and Rosenberg, I. (2010) 'Water, hydration, and health.' *Nutrition Reviews 68*(8), 439–458.

101. Natural Hydration Council (2014a) 'Hydration for children.' Hydration Fact Sheets. Available at www. naturalhydrationcouncil.org.uk/hydration-facts/fact-sheets/, accessed on 15 October 2014. Natural Hydration Council (2014b) 'Parents call for greater access to drinking water in primary schools.' Available at www.naturalhydrationcouncil.org.uk/press/parents-call-for-greater-access-to-drinking-water-in primary-schools/

102. Ibid.

103. Chaplin, M. (2006) 'Do we underestimate the importance of water in cell biology?' *Nature Reviews Molecular Cell Biology 7*(11), 861–866, p.861.

104. WHO (World Health Organization) (2005) *Nutrients in Drinking Water, Water, Sanitation and Health Protection and the Human Environment.* Geneva: WHO. Available at www.who.int/water_sanitation_health/dwq/nutrientsindw.pdf, accessed on 18 August 2015.

105. Ibid.

106. Kolodziejczyk, J., Flatt, S., Natarajan, L., Patterson, R., Pierce, J. and Norman, G. (2012) 'Associations of soluble fiber, whole fruits/vegetables, and juice with plasma Beta-carotene concentrations in a free-living population of breast cancer survivors.' *Women Health 52*(8), 731–743.

107. Sengupta, P. (2013) 'Potential health impacts of hard water.' *International Journal of Preventative Medicine 4*(8), 866.

108. Ahearn, W., Castine, T., Nault, K. and Green, G. (2001) 'An assessment of food acceptance in children with autism.' *Journal of Autism and Developmental Disorders 31*(5), 505–511.

109. Quoted in Cermak, S., Curtin, C. and Bandini, L. (2010) 'Food selectivity and sensory sensitivity in children with autism spectrum disorders.' *Journal of the American Dietetic Association 110*(2), 238–246, p.245.

110. Jean, A. (2001) 'Brain stem control of swallowing: neuronal network and cellular mechanisms.' *Physiological Reviews 81*(2), 929–969.

111. Palmieri, L. and Persico, A. (2010) 'Mitochondrial dysfunction in autism spectrum disorders: cause or effect?' *Biochimica et Biophysica Acta (BBA)-Bioenergetics 1797*(6), 1130–1137.

112. Kang, V., Wagner, G.C. and Ming, X. (2014) 'Gastrointestinal dysfunction in children with autism spectrum disorders.' *Autism Research 7*(4), 501–506. Lightdale, J., Gremse, D., Heitlinger, L., Cabana, M., Gilger, M. *et al.* (2013) 'Gastroesophageal reflux: management guidance for the pediatrician.' *Pediatrics 131*(5), e1684–e1695.

113. Schreck, K. A., Williams, K. and Smith, A. F. (2004) 'A comparison of eating behaviors between children with and without autism.' *Journal of Autism and Developmental Disorders 34*(4) 433–438.

114. Cermak, S A., Curtin, C. and Bandini, L.G. (2010) 'Food selectivity and sensory sensitivity in children with autism spectrum disorders.' *Journal of the American Dietetic Association 110*(2), 238–246.

115. Fraker, C., Fishbein, M., Cox, S. and Walbert, L. (2007) *Food Chaining: The Proven 6-Step Plan to Stop Picky Eating, Solve Feeding Problems and Expand Your Child's Diet.* Philadelphia, PA: Da Capo Press.

116. Ibid.

INDEX